CW00521009

The Vital Meridian
A Modern Exploration of Acupuncture

The cover character, 'Jing', which signifies 'meridian', is based on the Li Shu style of the calligrapher Han Ren Ming, who worked during the period of the Han Dynasty, 210BC–AD210. Drawn by Gabrielle Wang.

The Vital Meridian
A Modern Exploration of Acupuncture

Alan Bensoussan BSc Dip Ed Dip Ac C Ac (China)
Lecturer, School of Nursing and Health Studies,
University of Western Sydney (Macarthur)
Member, Council of the Sydney College of Traditional
Chinese Medicine

Foreword by
Giovanni Maciocia C Ac (Nanjing)
Acupuncturist and Medical Herbalist

CHURCHILL LIVINGSTONE
MELBOURNE EDINBURGH LONDON AND NEW YORK 1991

CHURCHILL LIVINGSTONE
Medical Division of Longman Group UK Limited

Distributed in Australia by Longman Cheshire Pty Limited, Longman House, King's Gardens, 95 Coventry Street, South Melbourne 3205, and by associated companies, branches and representatives throughout the world.

First published 1991

ISBN 0-443-04255-1

British Library Cataloguing in Publication Data
Bensoussan, Alan
  The vital meridian.
  1. Acupuncture
  I. Title
  615.892

Library of Congress Cataloging in Publication Data
Bensoussan, Alan.
  The vital meridian: a modern exploration of acupuncture/
Alan Bensoussan; foreword by Giovanni Maciocia.
  p.   cm.
  Includes index.
  ISBN 0-443-04255-1
  1. Acupuncture—Physiological aspects.   I. Title.
RM184.B45   1990
615.8'92—dc20   90-2114

Produced by Longman Singapore Publishers (Pte) Ltd
Printed in Singapore

Foreword

Acupuncture is a living and stubborn challenge to established 'scientific' knowledge. Its roots are at the very least 4000 years old and it is based on a philosophy and view of the body-mind that is entirely different from modern views. It is a total anachronism but it refuses to disappear. Of course, practitioners know that it 'works', that it is not 'in the mind' and that its mode of action can be 'explained' if only one accepts its conceptual premises. If Qi and channels really exist, then modern 'scientific' views of the body-mind clearly need to be revised. The problem is, of course, that acupuncture and the modern model of body-mind are different and spring from entirely different conceptual frameworks.

Up to now, there have been two quite distinct groups of people involved in acupuncture: on the one hand the practitioners of this 'art' who are, on the whole, quite unconcerned about explaining its mode of functioning in the light of modern science, and on the other hand, researchers who are not practitioners and whose only concern is to explain 'how it works' in the light of modern science. There is really very little communication between these two groups.

This book is the first attempt at bridging the gap between these two groups of people. It is the first book on the scientific aspects of acupuncture written by a practitioner. This makes it totally different from other books on the scientific aspects of acupuncture. Alan Bensoussan's exposition of the scientific views on the phenomena of channels and Qi is enriched and deepened by his experience as a practitioner. This is what makes his book so valuable and unique.

He makes accessible to acupuncture practitioners a large number of scientific studies that are relevant to our practice. It is also possible that the scope of acupuncture can be broadened as a result of such scientific studies.

This book will therefore be invaluable to practitioners and students of acupuncture who wish to familiarize themselves with the nature and breadth of research in acupuncture.

1991   Giovanni Maciocia

Acknowledgements

The motivation for this book came initially from discussions held in 1984 with Professor Mu Jian, a research physiologist at the Nanjing College of Traditional Chinese Medicine. His enthusiasm was welcomed and followed rapidly by my own extensive reading and preparation for a lecture course that I have held on contemporary acupuncture research at the New South Wales College of Traditional Chinese Medicine. I would like to thank both colleges for their support. A special word of thanks to Dr Peter Sheldon for his late night assistance on the computer, and of course, endless thanks to Sarah Loue and Emy.

Every effort has been made to trace copyright holders. The author and publishers would be pleased to hear from the owners of any copyright whom they have been unable to trace.

Contents

Introduction

Over the last 15 years acupuncture has dramatically increased in popularity as a therapy in most corners of the globe. So has the research that attempts to legitimate its use in terms of western science. However, few published articles or texts have appeared to date that review the scope and significance of these research findings. One exception to this is the outstanding work of Joseph Needham and Lu Gwen dju (1980), *Celestial Lancets: A History and Rationale of Acupuncture and Moxibustion*. This is one of the few publications I have read which explores with honesty and rigour the contemporary development of a scientific understanding of acupuncture.

To researchers acupuncture presents a specific problem in that it is a different scientific model from western medicine and adopts distinct terminology (such as 'energy' and 'channels'). This has constantly hindered communication between traditional Chinese doctors and orthodox medical practitioners. However, over the last two decades there has been a significant attempt to bridge the gap in terminology and experience by researching to understand three particular aspects of acupuncture science.

The first goal of research is to comprehend how diagnostic terminology may be equated (if at all) between Chinese and western medical paradigms. For example, could different tongue shapes, colours and coats have a meaningful interpretation in the western model? How can pulse qualities be accurately translated?

Secondly, researchers and clinicians have as a goal the identification of the potential and limitations of acupuncture. This is achieved by employing a substantial range of appropriately designed clinical studies. To the keen traditionalist it may appear somewhat repetitive and unnecessary in the light of the centuries of acupuncture experience in China. However, I hasten to add that clinical studies *are* providing us with fresh and promising possibilities for the application of acupuncture as we shall see in later chapters. Furthermore, with the arrival of 'new' illnesses such as acquired immune deficiency sydrome (AIDS) and myalgic encephalomyelitis (ME) and the existence of diseases foreign to China such as multiple sclerosis, we require some parameters by which to assess the clinical effectiveness of acupuncture in these cases.

The third goal of research has been to understand the mechanisms (in orthodox western terms) behind the workings of acupuncture. This direction of study is also appearing to enlarge upon the possible applications of acupuncture.

This text focuses particularly on the second and third research goals.

At the crudest level acupuncture is a technique of initiating, controlling or accelerating physiological functions of the body. But of course it extends far beyond this basic interpretation. Acupuncture theory incorporates a complete scientific model that permits the precise calculation of which acupuncture points to use, when and how to stimulate them, and which points to combine together—all based on observations of the symptoms and signs of the patient.

The theoretical paradigms that uphold the clinical practice of acupuncture are very different from western medical models. The oriental model appears to be more dependent upon the integration of a wide range of data, and a decision is seldom based on one or two factors alone. The fundamental reason for this is that no symptom or sign provides a single objective reading which acts as a basis for a diagnostic conclusion. In the Chinese model any piece of information (symptom or sign) gathered from the patient can only be interpreted subjectively in relation to other symptoms and signs. In other words any one observation on the patient may hold several meanings dependent upon other observations made of the patient. For example, a bright red tongue may be meaningfully interpreted as a full hot patient constitution if there is a thick yellow tongue coat and a strong pulse, or as a (yin) deficiency syndrome if the tongue coat is missing and the pulse is thin. The meaning of the red tongue is most clearly stated by observing other data.

The question must be asked, then, whether this subjective integration of patient data is useful in the management of illness (do not be fooled into thinking there are not strict guidelines for such integration). A clinical situation may be all that is needed to highlight this point. Imagine the scenario where two patients arrive at a general practice clinic both complaining of low back pain:

Patient A presents with a stiff and painful back especially after being seated for a while, or in the mornings upon rising. The patient feels better after a half hour or so of moving around and warmth seems to help;
Patient B registers worse back pain when he overworks. The pain tends to develop in the afternoon and goes on into the evening although is less severe on the weekends and rest seems to help.

In both patients X rays and blood tests show no abnormality. What would the general medical practitioner diagnose, and how would he or she act upon the diagnosis? If X rays and blood tests show no abnormality, are these cases necessarily distinct to the general practitioner?

In terms of the Chinese medical model they are quite different—in fact they represent opposite ends of a spectrum. Let me explain. Integral to the Chinese model is the concept of 'energy', which not only moves through the body, but ebbs and flows in different organs and regions of the body during the 24 hours of the day. Hence, to the Chinese not only does the blood circulate (and may I reiterate Joseph Needham's correction of the medical historians who still claim that William Harvey was the first to realise this) but so does 'vital energy', that is, the potential for physiological or mechanical activity, including the movement of blood.

So, pain after rest relates to poor circulation of this vital energy (at least) and maybe blood (if the situation is more severe). This pain responds to activation, to movement, which increases the flow of energy and clears the stagnation. On the other hand, pain associated with increased tiredness (that is, as the day goes on) and responds to rest, must be related to a deficiency or weakness of energy. Hence, in patient A the treatment is directed toward clearing the stagnation, that is, dispersing the build up or blockage, or in Chinese terms 'sedating an area of excess'. In patient B the treatment is directed toward building up and strengthening any areas of weakness, or in Chinese terms 'tonifying a deficiency'.

Clearly, these patients represent opposite ends of a spectrum and so does their management protocol. In this fashion the integration of the symptom, pain, with one other sign, the timing of pain, has provided useful clinical information for directing treatment with acupuncture, massage or Chinese herbs. Other symptoms and signs could have been explored to confirm these diagnostic findings.

In China there is an enormous amount of integration between the two systems (modern medicine and traditional Chinese medicine). In many hospitals a triage team assists the patient in selecting an appropriate form of treatment. The style of exchanges in information involve, for example, using modern diagnostic techniques followed by traditional Chinese therapies. As a specific example, ultrasound may be used for determining gallstone or kidney stone size and then, if appropriate, treatment may be given with acupuncture or herbs. Similarly, once it were ascertained (by employing modern diagnostic tools) that a presenting case of amenorrhea were due to a functional rather than organic disturbance, acupuncture might be a preferred form of therapy to contemporary hormonal drugs. In Australia there is less awareness of, and experience with, the potential of acupuncture among the medical profession.

Unfortunately, few western acupuncture researchers adequately review work that has previously been undertaken in their field of investigation. It almost appears as if each investigator were unveiling to the world a new and potent application, or interpretation, of acupuncture. This may also be a reflection of the fact that few of the authors writing on medical or scientific aspects of acupuncture possess sufficiently thorough training in the theory of Chinese medicine or the skills of this art.

There are many difficulties in producing a thorough review of acupuncture research. I have, in the introductory and final chapters, criticised the quality of some research work, but, of course, there has been an enormous amount of academic work which represents the major sources for this book. To review critically the tens of thousands of papers and research findings on acupuncture would require several volumes alone, and it is not the purpose of this text.

Hence, I have needed to be selective and have made qualitative judgements based upon:

1. Experimental technique. The research should be able to provide a valid measure of what it is purported to assess. It is important to note that the concepts being researched should be true to traditional Chinese medicine and not riddled with theoretical misconceptions from the start.

2. Endorsement of results by other researchers under similar or different conditions. The experiment should exhibit reliability.

It is impossible to cover everything. For example, I have excluded all research on other aspects of traditional Chinese medical theory and have concentrated solely on acupuncture. In doing so I have endeavoured to ensure that all areas of acupuncture research are covered.

Chapter 1 will explore contemporary acupuncture, particularly the fashion in which it has developed in the last decades, and its current role as a health care option. Chapter 2 investigates the physiological effects of acupuncture, especially of course, in biomedical terms. In Chapter 3 we are able to embark on the interesting findings of recent research on the acupuncture channels and points themselves. This touches new fields in medicine, and is picked up again in the closing chapter. Chapter 4 commences the review of research on neurophysiological mechanisms related to the workings of acupuncture. We explore how different systems are influenced, and this is taken up in further detail in Chapter 5.

This review of research is designed to equip the keen reader with some links and direction on the contemporary exploration of acupuncture. This text is in *no way an attempt to justify the practice of acupuncture*, for this would entail making enormous and impossible leaps between different medical models. It may, however, facilitate a field of intercommunication which, in turn, could only assist in the integration of Chinese medicine to the benefit of both clients and practitioners. I hope that by covering the major areas of acupuncture research it becomes a useful starting point for interested practitioners, researchers, readers and others.

1. Setting the scene of contemporary acupuncture

It is not uncommon to hear it said by practitioners and students of traditional Chinese medicine (TCM), as well as to read in popular texts, that the framework of TCM is sufficient in itself for successful application of this form of medical practice. This is often promoted as an argument against seeking explanations in western medical terms for the successes of acupuncture. Generally speaking, successful practice usually necessitates remaining true to a system and its boundaries but, as we shall see, it is just as important to comprehend how those boundaries are defined and what constitutes the 'system'.

In the case of traditional Chinese medicine a historical perspective of its growth patterns and practices may clarify its contemporary working context, and for this purpose detailed discussions are available in many texts.[1,2] As the following examples illustrate, modern acupuncture is distinctly different from the way it was practised 100 years ago, or many centuries prior to that. In some way our system or boundaries have changed, with the result that aspects we consider to be 'traditional' in Chinese medicine may, in fact, turn out not to be very 'traditional', nor in some cases, even 'Chinese'. In other instances the most fundamental clinical practices of TCM in Chinese hospitals are based upon modern exploration of acupuncture therapy.

Scalp acupuncture, for example, has been properly developed only since 1970, and even then only on the basis of knowledge of localisation of brain function according to orthodox western medicine.[3,4] As points are located and named in conformation with cerebral functional areas, the principal indications for scalp needling are neurological in nature.[5,6] Scalp acupuncture has no 'traditional' development in TCM, it is certainly difficult to integrate it thoroughly with acupuncture channel theory, and it evades easy explanation even in the broader context of TCM theory. Yet it boasts a significant role in the management of neuromuscular disorders (e.g., sensory and motor paralysis) and psychiatric diseases.[7]

Similarly, ear acupuncture has been a serious concern only since Nogier's work in 1957 in Europe.[8] Prior to that there is brief mention in the *Nei Jing*, (the Yellow Emperor's classic of internal medicine), and other classics such as the *Zhen Jiu Da Cheng* (Compendium of acupuncture and moxibustion), although nothing which has resulted in its adoption as an important form of treatment. Clearly, ear acupuncture also lacks any distinct path of traditional development and now requires certain a flexibility when using it in the context of TCM theory. By way of example, many points have western medical names and are selected with western physiological concepts in mind, such as the endocrine point for menstrual disorders, or the sympathetic nerve point for circulatory disorders or muscular spasms.[9]

When we consider other branches of acupuncture therapy, we discover that in the 1960s acupuncture anaesthesia experienced a surge in popularity amongst researchers, if not their patients. This was also a very new application for acupuncture. Although the analgesic properties of acupuncture have been well known for centuries, particularly in the context of treating painful disorders such as headaches and arthritis, it was not until 1958 in Shanghai that the first surgical operations were performed under acupuncture anaesthesia. This occurred following successful trials on postoperative pain. The technique of acupuncture anaesthesia is therefore founded on relatively new experience, and once again we observe that a branch of acupuncture has negligible roots in the history of TCM theory. This is particularly so when we consider the most important and successful analgesic points (for surgery) are on the ear. (It is important to state, however, that some points for anaesthesia are selected using traditional channel theory.)[10]

It is not only the techniques of scalp and ear acupuncture, and acupuncture anaesthesia that are recent developments in TCM. Although empirical observations have formed the building blocks of TCM theory over the centuries, many clinical procedures and treatments are based specifically on the outcome of contemporary clinical research.

As an example, the points Fuliu (Kid 7), and Yinxi (Ht 6) are a common prescription for night sweats. Some justification for their use may be provided by TCM theory, however this formula was the outcome of clinical research.[11] Similarly, the points Houxi (SI 3), Weizhong (Bl 40), Tianzhu (Bl 10), Renzhong (Du 26) and the lumbago point on the back of the hand are often used for back pain, depending upon its location. The selection (in the Jiangsu District TCM Hospital) of a suitable point is based upon TCM theory as well as reports of research results.[12] Another example is the superior use of Renying (St. 9) for hypertension, also a consequence of recent investigation.

The routine selection of these popular acupuncture points illustrates the clinical importance of undertaking research, as they have each in turn added in some way to the scope and efficacy of acupuncture. It would appear that modern research has already contributed in a significant manner to the development of traditional Chinese medicine.

Incorporation of electricity and laser to stimulate acupuncture points is a further example of the shifts in the boundaries of the TCM system. Microwave acupuncture is another more recent example. It has been used experimentally to boost the immunological function of cancer patients.[13] Although earlier texts assert that obtaining Qi sensation is of vital importance in successful acupuncture treatment, stimulation of points with laser achieves no Qi sensation whatsoever. Hence, with the incorporation of laser, successsful or not, we have moved away from maintaining the important parameters and therefore the theoretical concepts paramount in the TCM model.

Returning briefly to the examples of scalp and ear acupuncture we cannot even claim that in these cases, as we are using needles but placing them in different loci, we are still being traditional. The obvious danger here is that we are separating and isolating the concept of 'needles' or 'stimulation loci' from that of 'channel theory'. One developed hand in hand with the other, and to adopt one concept without the other is to break up the unity and consistency of the theoretical fabric of Chinese medicine. Our sticking of needles elsewhere is no longer 'traditional acupuncture'. After all, the theory of traditional Chinese medicine has always guided the selection of points for various illnesses, and equally emphasised the importance of needle technique.

This calls to mind an encounter I once had with a Greek man who was managing a local milkbar near my clinic in York, England. In his youth back home he was viewed as a local healer, adopting many of the ancient and traditional medical skills of Greece. Amongst the many events in his past, he related an episode whereby he claimed to have saved the life of a fellow villager who was experiencing severe cardiac pain, by slashing his earlobe. Tall story or not, letting blood from the ear is a traditional technique even in Chinese medicine. For example, *Acupuncture: A Comprehensive Text*[14] claims, 'there are prescriptions in traditional folk medicine for treating redness of the eye by pricking the ear lobes or by letting blood from the posterior auricular vein in the treatment of pain and redness in the eye.'(p 472) However, something would be amiss if, on the basis of this Greek man's story, practitioners began slashing various other extremities in the hope that a whole range of illnessses would be cured.

It is not to say that this technique will not work, although, like sticking pins in new regions in the scalp or ear, supplementing them with electric current or laser, or choosing points for reasons other than traditional theory, it initially has no empirical or scientific foundation.

Nevertheless, certain techniques are eventually adopted into the gamut of TCM. This is principally because they have established their status in recent medical history as a consequence of clinical research, and present themselves as successful and justifiable choices for therapy. Hence, some major approaches mentioned earlier, though not traditional, are employed today as a result of recent research. Bearing this in mind, it is clear that contemporary students and practitioners of acupuncture must not only modify their claims of traditionality and 'centuries of medical experience', but also become familiar with the outcomes of this research. It would appear that much of what is learnt clinically in China and overseas is the 'new' traditional Chinese medicine.

On modern acupuncture research

As contemporary acupuncture practice is in part the result of ongoing research, it is important to review ways in which this research has been able to work toward improving the clinical effectiveness of acupuncture therapy. As acupuncturists, our initial question is how do we go about studying and researching TCM to improve our clinical skill? In the following I hope to illustrate how imperative it is to possess a good sense of the characteristics of acupuncture and TCM theory in order to carry out valuable research. More specifically, it is important to have a good sense of TCM theory in order to know what questions to formulate for research.

Knowledge of TCM is all about having a good understanding of the characteristics of the system and how it works in a practical sense. For example, we need to be aware of the relationship between the nature of disease and the treatment modality selected, that is, the effect of a treatment may depend on the nature of the presenting disease. As a specific example, in herbal medicine, Da Huang (rhubarb) may be used not only for constipation, but also for diarrhea, depending upon the nature of the illness (hot/cold), and the dosage of rhubarb. In hypertension, Renying (St 9) is the most successful acupuncture point empirically, but more important in Shi (Excess) than Xu (Deficient) cases. Therefore simply to diagnose hypertension and use Renying (St 9) may not be suitable treatment. Similarly, we know from our own clinical experience that needle technique is crucial, and that results may vary according to the patient's constitution, the presenting disease, and the needle technique selected.

Unfortunately, from a review of international report documents, it is clear that many researchers possess insufficient background in Chinese medicine. They have a poor feeling for its characteristics and may not be in a position to formulate appropriate (research) questions. Consequently many research papers from the West (and a considerable number from the East) contain many fallacies and misunderstandings of TCM. Let me explain this further.

When researchers construct questions, they already have a theory in mind which needs testing, and they usually have definite preconceptions that allow them to formulate the questions. The very act of question construction demands some background information. In order to design questions researchers will have already made certain observations, which inevitably will have been also interpreted in some existing ideology. Specifically, researchers need to avoid excessive ideology in framing their questions for investigation.

The questions asked at the outset of research are of paramount importance because they will often determine the outcome. In fact, as I demonstrate in subsequent chapters, research has shown that acupuncture may bring about almost any possible physiological effect, provided the research question is directed in a nominated way. The failure of such research is that it has not assisted in defining anything new, such as the boundaries of acupuncture practice. It has only provided proof in answer to a question upon which an opinion had already been formed. There was already a hunch that such a physiological effect would be likely, based on information from clinical experience. (Partly because of the enormous numbers of papers with differing experimental boundaries and measurement techniques, some researchers arrive at contradictory findings. This is not new in any of the sciences. Brian Martin in *The Bias of Science* provides one of the most outstanding analyses of how this may occur.)[15]

For example, assume we wish to know whether needling particular acupuncture points brings about dilation or constriction of the blood vessels. We may consider this important as it would lead to a change in total peripheral resistance, and consequently affect cardiac output and mean arterial blood pressure. In answer to our question, *Acupuncture: A Comprehensive Text*[14] reports on some experiments stating, 'Measurements taken on the fingers and ears showed that needling Hegu (Co 4) and Waiguan (SJ 5) caused vasodilation, while needling Neiguan (Pe 6) caused vasoconstriction'(p 532).

How would we design an experiment to measure and confirm this? In doing so, what variables or factors would we need to neglect or eliminate? What may be surprising is that no matter what experiment we design to address this question, if we repeated it a few times we would be likely to find that our results differ markedly each time. Why? Because the question itself shows insufficient understanding of TCM. Traditional Chinese medicine has never claimed needling specifically causes vasoconstriction or vasodilation, or that this is one way acupuncture works, or that it will help us understand how it works. Yet the question shows good understanding of modern physiology, as needling will stimulate nerve endings causing a sympathetic response of vasoconstriction or vasodilation. Experienced acupuncturists could say that vasoconstriction or vasodilation may depend upon:

1. A person's health and constitution at the time. (Yang xu, yin xu, hot/cold, sweating or not, fever or not, blood pressure up or down, etc. Each of these categories describes the presence of certain symptoms and signs which are deemed, according to TCM theory, to be relevant to the outcome of treatment.)
2. The time of needling. (Day/night, open hourly points, season, weather conditions—all generally related to cycles of Qi.)
3. The needle technique. (Cooling the heavens [tou tian liang], setting mountain on fire [shao shan huo], the depth of needling, tonifying and reducing, enhancement of needle sensation with Qi Gong, etc.)

These factors are part of traditional Chinese medical theory, and they are also a simple statement that certain parameters are significant in predicting the outcome of needling. Hence they require consideration during the selection of points for an acupuncture prescription. The truth of such aspects of traditional clinical theory is increasingly confirmed by experimental research.[16]

It is not surprising that the Shanghai text[14] goes on to state in the same paragraph:

Concerning the influence of acupuncture on vasoconstriction and vasodilation and the rules by which this is governed, reports differ. Most of the evidence suggests that acupuncture lowers the degree of tension and relaxes the walls of blood vessels in patients with high levels of vasoconstriction. When the tension is too low, acupuncture induces an increase in tension and vasoconstriction.... It was discovered that needling at different depths with varying intensities of stimulation brought different results.

Therefore, is the original question, attempting to determine which points are vasoconstrictive or vasodilatory, appropriate and useful in order to further our clinical skills in TCM? The results of experiments show we cannot find a consistent answer, which implies we need to redefine the question. How did we end up with such an inappropriate question? Because the question was asked in ignorance of factors which have already been shown *in clinical experience* to be of importance. And it was asked with a modern physiological framework in mind. With a new degree of awareness it will be necessary now to abandon this type of question completely and design a new style of question. However, before doing so, it may be worthwhile examining in more detail why these problems of definition and question construction occur when preparing to undertake research. Further insights are available if we inspect the nature of measurement and research.

Scientific research incorporates, in part, the measurement of variables to test the accuracy of a particular hypothesis. The act of taking measurements of a specific variable is in itself an act of focusing in on a particular site of action. For example, we may measure peripheral blood circulation (and hence an expression of vasoconstriction and vasodilation) by measuring microtemperature changes at the ear or fingertips. Measurements here have a very specific spatial and temporal focus. Furthermore, during the process of focusing in, the measurement techniques themselves require that as many other variables as possible be eliminated in order to maintain the accuracy of readings and evaluate the correctness or otherwise of our original hypothesis. In the case of microtemperature changes we may need to control, for example, excitement, weather, exercise, breathing, sleep, digestion and many more variables, all of which may influence our readings. In actuality though, it seems these variables are neglected rather than consciously controlled.

If anything is paramount in TCM theory, however, it is the integration and consideration of all significant variables that relate to the process of diagnosis and treatment. The design of treatment principles based on the integration of individual patient data is essential to the successful outcome of the treatment. Therefore it is the inescapable task of the good researcher to be aware of when some variables become significant, and when not. These need to be structured into the experimental design. Hence, the very nature of TCM theory and practice (to integrate variables) may be in direct conflict with the nature and method of current scientific research techniques (to control and eliminate variables). This conflict does not have to continue, especially if researchers become more informed about TCM, and the design and thinking behind experimentation alters.

The design of control groups, which variables we consider, and which we do not, and why, are all issues that may depend very much on the amount of

TCM knowledge researchers possess, and how they are able to incorporate that into their research procedure. Simple questions such as 'Can acupuncture control urinary bleeding, or can it control dysentery?' may end up being more fruitful and definite than the style of our earlier question 'Does acupuncture cause vasodilation or vasoconstriction?'. Importantly, the former question does not assume any physiological framework for testing the hypothesis. What it does assume, however, is the language to describe the pathological signs.

Although perhaps we can describe categories of treatment approaches, we must also allow acupuncture flexibility in the management of individual cases of haematuria (urinary bleeding). The points selected and needle techniques may both need to be varied in order to treat any presenting case successfully. Each case is not necessarily, or even likely to be, identical to the previous ones in Chinese diagnostic terms. Hence we can see that a certain flexibility is needed in order to measure accurately the usefulness of acupuncture, because of the very fact that the theory of acupuncture is structured around the integration of data. We would be failing in our research if we were to eliminate these variables, and as a result decide on a few acupuncture points, and needle these on everyone with haematuria.

Ideology behind question formation is even more significant in research into acupuncture *mechanisms*. Preconceptions guide the creation of questions and hypotheses that require testing. What we know may limit the ways we explore what we do not know.

When researchers explore a possible mechanism behind an observed treatment effect, they conceptualise backwards with the tools they possess and attempt to understand the process along known physiological pathways, that is, they investigate within the comfort of their own scientific confines. Acupuncture anaesthesia therefore would have to be mediated by nerves and neurotransmitters because that is the understood physiological mechanism behind analgesia.

This pattern of thinking is one reason why whatever we set out to look for we find. This reflects poorly on the sum total of research work, and makes a clear statement about its lack of direction. Acupuncture is known to bring about a wide spectrum of changes, that is, it has been clinically observed to treat a large number of conditions (see Table 2.3). Hence, an enormous number of effects may be recorded, and each, as a consequence of our research mentality, would be closely related to a specific, yet different, hypothesis.

Because the results of most research into acupuncture mechanisms are positive (that is, the opening hypothesis of the research is confirmed), we still possess no guidelines within which to comprehend the Chinese theoretical system. It may not come as a surprise then, that any hypothesis so far proposed by researchers to explain how acupuncture works fails in a significant sense, because none of these theories can be used to *predict* the outcome of needling any particular selection of acupuncture points. It is in this way that the research fails to define the boundaries of traditional acupuncture theory, an ancient theory that stakes a significant claim on its ability to predict the outcome of needling.

It would appear necessary to test beyond our conventional belief system in order to find these boundaries. More adventurous work is undertaken in some Eastern bloc countries and will be explored in Chapter 3. The work of people such as Reichmannis, Marino and Becker in exploring the nature of the channels ventures far away from the daily conventions of neurophysiology with the refreshing outcome of developing a bioelectric paradigm with which to understand the channels.[17,18,19]

Partly as a consequence of the failure of research to define the working boundaries of acupuncture, various theories have been proposed to explain its actions. The very fact that so many theories exist is clearly indicative that any one theory offered so far is incapable of accounting for all the facets of acupuncture therapy. Although this reflects poorly on each theory, there are many scientific phenomena that have been explained using dual theories. For example, the behaviour of light may best be explained by using the concept of energy quanta in some instances, or wave motion in others, depending upon the experimental circumstances and the ease with which either descriptive analogy may be adopted. Yet for some time a reverse argument has been used to justify why acupuncture should *not* be incorporated into the armoury of medical institutions, that is, because more than one theory may be used to explain its effects. (Mankind still uses light, even though scientists do not completely understand it.)

On the adoption of acupuncture into the western medical system

Of course incomplete scientific explanation does not negate the existence of a phenomenon, nor does it preclude it from practical use. Restricting our discussion to the context of health care, many medicines and medical procedures that have been and are presently used are applied without a knowledge of their precise mechanism or principles of operation. There is no need to search far to find that a fair proportion of what we consider to be 'proven' scientifically falls considerably short of our expectations. Standard drug manuals reveal this for many commonly employed drugs. To cite just a couple from the Physician's Desk Manual.[20]

Librium (sedative): The precise mechanism of action is not known.(p 1512)
Motrin (anti−inflammatory): Its mode of action, like that of other non−steroidal anti−inflammatory agents, is not known.(p 1854)

The following quotation from Jonathon Wright's *The Satisfactions and Frustrations of Nutritional Medicine*[21] also contains an example:

A congressional report (Office of Technology Assessment, U.S. Congress, Assessing the Efficacy of Medical Technology, 1978) concludes that only 10 to 20 percent of present-day 'scientific' medical procedures have been shown, by controlled clinical trial, to be of benefit. One possible interpration of this congressional document is that 80 to 90 percent of modern scientific medicine has no better scientific proof behind it than snake oil.

Electroconvulsive therapy (ECT) is also an example of a medical procedure that is still in use in psychiatric hospitals today despite the fact that very little is known about it.

Hence, without overshadowing the enormous efforts (and expenditure of vast sums of money), particular aspects of commonly adopted medications and techniques currently evade explanation. On the other hand, as we shall see in the following chapters, ample clinical studies have been carried out throughout the world to show that acupuncture is a highly effective form of treatment. Acupuncture research certainly matches up both in quality and in quantity when compared with some of the research on drugs and medical procedures that are routinely employed.

As pointed out by Robyn Williams, an eminent science journalist with the Australian Broadcasting Corporation, 'We simply can't wait until medical research has satisfied itself that the proof is in and the case closed. For a start, such conclusive proof is *never* established [my emphasis].'[22] (p 102)

It is also important to note that TCM theory is a formulation of concepts based upon empirical observation and research. It may be considered an approximation of what happens in reality just like many scientific theories, and consequently is true only under certain conditions. But in the growth of TCM theory we have witnessed a conscientious adoption of scientific principles. The study of Chinese medical history reveals that theories have been altered and built upon using scientific methodology specifically by:

1. Making clinical observations;
2. Systematising these observations into theory;
3. Verifying these theories by further testing and observation; and
4. Modifying original theories in the light of new information.

The diligent adoption of these scientific principles over the millennia carries a strong argument in favour of the 'science' of Chinese medical theory — different as it is to our own.

The lack of safety in the act of acupuncture has also been propounded as an argument against its adoption and popularisation. However, this also begs to be placed in the context of the hazards presented by some current drugs and procedures. For example, reporting on a study conducted at a Boston hospital and published in the *New England Journal of Medicine*, Steel et al state[23] 'We found that (290) 36% of 815 consecutive patients on a general medical service of a university hospital had an iatrogenic illness. In 9% of all persons admitted, the incident was considered major in that it threatened life or produced considerable disability.' (p 638) Furthermore 2% died because of their treatment.

In a similar study doctors found 36 operating room mistakes among 5 612 patients[24] 'In two thirds of the cases the mishap was due to . . . an unnecessary, defective or inappropriate operative procedure. In eleven [patients] death was directly attributable to the error.' (p 634) The mistakes added an average 42 days to their stays in hospital at a combined cost of over $1.7 million. Clearly, the risks incurred during hospitalisation are not trivial.

Even harsher statistics are provided by Ivan Illich[25] and other authors. Kennith Pelletier states in *Holistic Medicine*[26]

Recently, a congressional report from a subcommittee of the U.S. House of Representatives announced a disturbing fact. They concluded from their investigations that 2.4 million unnecessary surgical procedures were performed in 1974 at a cost of 4 billion dollars. Even of greater concern is the fact that these unnecessary surgeries resulted in 11 900 deaths.

Issues of safety and scientific method aside, ultimately the encouragement of medical and scientific exploration of traditional Chinese medicine will lead to the creation of a field of communication between the two sciences. It will provide future practitioners with increased understanding of the two models, and increased ease of crossreferral. For the benefit of patients it will also expose new vistas of possibility in the management of a multitude of disorders.

Examination of modern medical procedures through the eyes of the TCM model may similarly produce advantageous results. For example, in seeking an understanding of acute and chronic anxiety, practitioners, by adopting traditional Chinese diagnosis, are often guided to the use of tonifying treatments in acupuncture and herbs to support and nourish the body. This represents a significantly different approach to modern medicine's employment of sedatives to numb the mind. Such sharing of clinical experience seems certain to highlight new options for patient management.

Fresh approaches to therapy are one healthy outcome of the successful cross-fertilisation of these two medical paradigms. This duality, a consequence of global cultural exchange, represents nothing less than a scientific gift to a generation of practitioners. What a disservice it would be to squander the opportunity to engage each medical option to the fullest. New approaches can only be a reality with increased communication across our medical paradigms. Clinical and experimental studies are one step toward bridging that scientific and theoretical chasm.

REFERENCES

1. Wang K C, Wu L T 1973 (orig. 1932) History of Chinese medicine. AMS Press, New York
2. Unschuld P U 1985 Medicine in China: a history of ideas. University of California Press, London
3. Shi Y 1984 Lecture on the occasion of the fourth international advanced acupuncture studies program. Nanjing College of Traditional Chinese Medicine, China
4. Lu H (trans) 1975 Scalp acupuncture: therapy and anaesthesia. Academy of Oriental Heritage, Vancouver
5. Liu T H, Sadove M S 1974 Scalp needle therapy—acupuncture treatment for central nervous disorders. American Journal of Chinese Medicine 2(3): 261—269

6. Shi Z, Gong B, Jia Y, Huo Z 1987 The efficacy of electroacupuncture on 98 cases of epilepsy. Journal of Traditional Chinese Medicine 7(1): 21–22
7. Zhang M J 1985 Nanjing Neuropsychiatric Institute, Personal communication
8. Nogier P M F 1980 Handbook to auriculotherapy. (Kenyon J trans) Maisoneuve, Paris
9. Huang H L (trans) 1974 Ear acupuncture. Rodale Press, Pennsylania
10. Needham J, Lu G 1980 Celestial lancets: a history and rationale of acupuncture and moxibustion. Cambridge University Press, Cambridge
11. Wu X, 1985 Nanjing College of Traditional Chinese Medicine, Personal communication
12. Chen Z, Zhou X 1984 The effect of acupuncture in 300 cases of acute lumbar sprain. Journal of Traditional Chinese Medicine 4(2): 93–95
13. He C, Gong K, Xu Q, Yu Y, Liang H, Gu F 1987 Effects of microwave acupuncture on the immunological function of cancer patients. Journal of Traditional Chinese Medicine 7(1): 9–11
14. Shanghai College of Traditional Chinese Medicine 1983 Acupuncture: a comprehensive text. O'Connor J and Bensky D (trans). Eatsland Press, Chicago
15. Martin B 1979 The bias of science. Society for Social Responsibility in Science, Canberra
16. Chen K, Liang S, Feng X 1984 The effect of acupuncture using reinforcing and reducing methods on nail microcirculation and local skin temperature. Journal of Traditional Chinese Medicine 4(4): 279–281
17. Reichmannis M, Marino A A, Becker R O 1975 Electrical correlates of acupuncture points. Institute of Electrical and Electronics Transactions on Biomedical Engineering. Nov: 533–535
18. Reichmannis M, Marino A A, Becker R O 1976 DC skin conductance variation at acupuncture loci. American Journal of Chinese Medicine 4(1): 69–72
19. Becker R O 1974 The basic biological transmission and control system influenced by electrical forces. Annals of the New York Academy of Science 238: 236–241
20. Physician's Desk Manual 1986 ER Barnhart, New Jersey
21. Wright J V 1983 The satisfactions and frustrations of nutritional medicine. Rodale Press, Pennsylvania
22. Williams R 1987 Outpourings. Penguin, Melbourne
23. Steel K, Gertman P M, Cresscenzi C, Anderson J 1981 Iatrogenic illness on a general medical service at a university hospital. New England Journal of Medicine 304(11): 638–641
24. Couch N P, Tilney N L, Rayner A A, Moore F D 1981 The high cost of low frequency events, the anatomy and economics of surgical mishaps. New England Journal of Medicine 304(11): 634–637
25. Illich I 1984 Limits to medicine. Penguin, Harmondsworth
26. Pelletier K R 1980 Holistic medicine. Delacorte Press, New York

FURTHER READING

Chalmers A 1979 What is this thing called science? University of Queensland Press, Brisbane
Hillier S M, Jewell J A 1983 Health care and traditional medicine in china 1800–1982. Routledge & Kegan Paul, London
Jayasuriya A 1981 Acupuncture science. Acupuncture Foundation of Sri Lanka, Sri Lanka
Lampton D M 1977 The politics of medicine in china. Westview Press, Colorado

2. The physiological effects of acupuncture

Can you treat low blood pressure?
My red blood cell count is supposed to be low. Can acupuncture help?
Are you able to help me control my blood sugar level/cholesterol level?.

These sorts of questions from patient to acupuncturist are not uncommon in the West. And they launch us straight into making crosscultural or, more specifically, cross-scientific judgements. Are TCM practitioners equipped to answer such questions even with their basic medical sciences background? Surely they are not just being asked to understand modern medical terms but also to correlate the language and theory of TCM and the language and theory of modern medicine. After all TCM practitioners do not diagnose 'low blood pressure', or 'low red blood cell count', or 'altered blood sugar, or cholesterol levels', all of which are meaningless terms to the TCM practitioner.

As acupuncturists is it necessary to answer these questions? Should we ignore them and respond with a 'sometimes' or 'maybe'. After all, how sure are we of what the answers to these questions depend upon? And, of course, we do have our TCM diagnosis to get on with!

Certainly, a large proportion of clients may be satisfied with no information (they trust you implicitly) or, on the other hand, they may be more than satisfied with, and interested in, the TCM interpretation. However, just as many may also be curious to know what to expect from the treatment in terms of their presenting pathological disorder, a concept they are already more likely to be familiar with, and understand, as a consequence of their cultural upbringing. Unquestionably, providing clients with information will assist in obtaining their compliance, not only for the course of treatment, but in making any imperative lifestyle adjustments (indicated by traditional Chinese medical theory).

Throughout China and in isolated pockets elsewhere, there is ample evidence of a push toward the integration of the two medical systems. It pervades many areas of medical practice, such as in diagnosis (for example, cholelithiasis is diagnosed definitively with ultrasound but often treated with acupuncture) and in surgical anaesthesia, where drugs (sedatives and mild analgesics) can be used in conjunction with acupuncture analgesia (AA) to augment the effect of AA, and therefore assist with patients in a high risk category for full drug anaesthesia.[1] Steps toward the integration of the two systems are also seen in some surgical procedures. For example, puncturing Suliao (Du 25) has been shown to assist fibrogastroscopic examination by relieving gastric hyperperistalsis and pyloric constriction, and associated nausea or retching.[2,3] In some treatments acupuncture is adopted in conjunction with other (drug) therapies in order to enhance their effects.[4] In the treatment of various cancers, Xia Yuqing et al, at the China Academy of TCM in Beijing, determined that acupuncture provided increased tolerance with substantially decreased side effects to patients undergoing radio- and chemotherapy, compared to a non-acupunctured control group. Similar results were observed in Russia in the treatment of edema of the extremities following radiation or combination therapy of cancer of the breast and uterus.[141]

Successful integration requires that meaningful dialogue be established between the two systems. Comparative studies are one way toward the establishment of this dialogue amongst practitioners on either side of the fence. Clients also benefit from increased communication with the practitioner and better management of the presenting condition.

In this chapter we will explore physiological changes to the body that are brought about by needling. These changes include metabolic changes and alterations of pathophysiology. The studies reviewed do provide the practitioner with the ability to respond more fruitfully to patients' questions.

As acupuncturists and TCM practitioners we do not need to be concerned at the likelihood of being swallowed up by orthodox medicine, a fear many practitioners no doubt share, should this path of integration be followed to completion. This is because contrasting scientific paradigms arise and develop out of different needs and cultural backgrounds — ultimately different frames of reference. Just as we have one medical paradigm that accounts for the concept of 'life force' (Qi), so we have another that describes the significance of hydroxycorticosteroids in the urine. Each has an important role to play that cannot be usurped by the other.

Health care situations will arise where the concept of 'life force' integrated into a medical framework of diagnosis and treatment will provide a solution to a problem not otherwise solvable using the biomedical paradigm. For example, the symptom of lethargy is particularly meaningful in the Chinese paradigm because it may be directly related to a disturbance of Qi and ultimately specific organ dysfunction. Through the concept of Qi, the therapist is able to arrive at a diagnosis and successful treatment. The western medical model however cannot class lethargy as any specific physiological disturbance and, if unsuccessful in finding a definite pathology (such as glandular fever), is often at a loss in treating such a debility.

Other occasions will arise where the TCM framework offers little support compared with the less subjective approach of modern medicine. For example, in the case of a comatosed, insulin dependent diabetic no amount of Chinese diagnosis or needling could replace the injection of insulin as a life saver.

But it is not our purpose here to discuss which medical system is most appropriate for any particular disease. Answers to such questions still await the accumulation of experience, both in China and elsewhere. For even China suffered from the relative isolation and separation of traditional and modern practitioners until the last two decades.

There are many different ways of approaching the discussion of the physiological effects of needling[5] (p 529-543), but in this chapter the following four broad areas are treated individually:

1. The analgesic effect of needling;
2. The regulatory effect of needling;
3. The ability to raise the defence and immunity of the organism;
4. The sedative and psychological effect of needling. Here we discuss the genuine psychological effects of acupuncture, and not the placebo response. The placebo response will be addressed separately in Chapter 4.

THE ANALGESIC EFFECT OF NEEDLING

In this section we will review the use of acupuncture for the management of painful disorders as well as its adoption in surgery as a form of analgesia. The general characteristics related to acupuncture analgesia (AA) in surgery will also be presented.

For over two decades and particularly during the last, an enormous amount of energy has been invested in exploring AA. This is for several reasons. Firstly, the popularisation of acupuncture in the West came about principally through observation of operations under AA in China. This sparked off more research in the field, both in the West, where enlightened physicians considered it to be acupuncture's forte, and in China, where the Chinese could see that more scientific research in AA would clearly assist the proliferation of its medicine in the West.

Secondly, exploring AA in surgery may lead to an understanding of the basis of acupuncture, which in turn may be helpful in the management of other disorders. Any applications of acupuncture would be assumed to share neural pathways as their mode of influence. Comprehending the neural basis of AA may help to shed light on how other physiological changes are brought about with acupuncture.

Finally, the induction of analgesia for surgery with acupuncture is a popular area for study because it can be observed immediately, and there is no need to consider relapses, remissions, uncertainty and psychosomatic influences, all more relevant in management of general disorders.

As we are talking about pain relief, it is worthwhile exploring the nature of pain within TCM before we proceed much further. In particular, it may be fruitful to contrast the diagnosis and subsequent management of pain in TCM with the treatment of pain by acupuncturists who do not use traditional Chinese medical theory. The latter is rather more symptomatic and simplistic.

This is very important because there is a discrepancy between the term 'pain relief' in TCM and modern medicine. In TCM relieving pain refers to the actual treatment of the disorder, not analgesia, because pain is always associated with a disorder, be that even, in Chinese terms, poor circulation of Qi and Blood.

In Chinese medicine, pain may be classified as Xu (deficient) or Shi (excess), where Shi generally represents the most painful conditions (i.e., stagnations of Qi and Blood, and stagnation due to Cold, which is especially painful). Xu pain may be a result of insufficient nourishment of Qi and Blood, or the Zangfu (organs and tissues), which results in the retardation of circulation of Qi and Blood. Common causative factors of pain in TCM include (where Xu and Shi aspects may be combined):

1. Stagnation of Qi
2. Stagnation of Blood
3. Accumulation of Cold
4. Accumulation of Heat
5. Retention of Phlegm.

Many pathogenic factors may lead to these five classes of painful syndromes, all of which, with a good understanding of TCM, may be beneficially treated by acupuncture. Relieving pain in Chinese terms may involve, for example, clearing Blood stagnation, as in thrombosis pain; clearing Qi stagnation, as in peripheral vascular problems (e.g., Raynaud's syndrome or thromboangeitis obliterans); or clearing accumulation of Heat, as in cystitis. Strangely enough, the diversity of ways in which acupuncture may relieve pain has not been credited by orthodox medical researchers, yet modern medicine itself manages pain wherever posssible through a better understanding of the disease rather than by just activating neurological blocks. Ischaemic heart pain, gastric ulcer pain and rheumatic inflammatory disorders are all managed with different drugs, even though each drug still has an influence on a neurological level. Unfortunately, medical researchers too often still claim that acupuncture brings about pain relief only via neurological blocks (including feedback cycles) rather than, for example, relaxing vascular constriction, or reducing gastric acids.[6]

When exploring the propensity of acupuncture to relieve pain, the Chinese did not just have the mobilisation of a neural effect as the purpose of treatment. *They also viewed with importance the need to address the central condition causing pain.* Correct acupuncture, properly directed to the management of pain, will also increase oxygenation of cardiac muscle, reduce gastric acidity, and control inflammatory responses. As we shall see in subsequent chapters, a vast number of neural and hormonal systems are involved in the modulation of pain.[7,8] The same hormonal and neural systems are also involved in physiological changes other than the reduction of pain.

The Chinese have always talked about clearing the presenting condition rather than simply dulling the area and possibly masking the disorder. An inclination towards the latter, unfortunately, is one outcome of the direction that research into AA has taken, because few researchers have been willing to explore the implications of needling beyond the targeted analgesic response that they are measuring.

A good understanding of TCM is necessary in order to be able to treat pain successfully with acupuncture. Simple knowledge of local, distal or empirical points, or treating by the meridian pathways alone is insufficient, according to traditional teaching. Chinese doctors claim lack of knowledge will greatly limit the success of the treatment, precisely because to treat pain related to the accumulation of heat, for example, requires specific points to be piqued, specific needle techniques ('cooling like a clear night sky'), or even more general techniques (such as bleeding the Jingwell points, or using moxa for the purpose of drawing fire away). If this condition were treated with a standard points prescription for pain in that region, then benefit may or may not occur, and certainly treatment would not be as effective. In general, certain points need to be selected instead of others because they have the empirical function of clearing Heat, Phlegm, Cold, or moving Blood and Qi. Otherwise, in the simplistic 'Fuliu (Kid 7) for knee pain' approach, we would be ignorant of large areas of the empirical development of TCM theory. The ancient fabric of theory has been woven with the innumerable threads of empirical observation. A good practitioner needs to look beyond the pattern of dyes on the material, and study the way the threads are woven together.

Hence, a crucial criterion by which to assess the quality of research work into the analgesic or pain relieving nature of acupuncture is to ensure that the research procedure includes a correct differentiation of the presenting cases using traditional Chinese medical principles. Only then can we be confident that we are on the road to incorporating acupuncture properly, and that we are likely to witness the genuine benefit of acupuncture. Even the experience of the practitioner is crucial here, as the needle technique, direction of Qi sensation, duration and frequency of treatment, point selection and location, and many other factors will all have an influence on the success of treatment. Naturally these expectations of research would apply not only to work done with analgesia, but to all the physiological effects of acupuncture.

Some papers manifest awareness of TCM by incorporating a TCM diagnosis into their research design. Subjects are individually diagnosed using Chinese medical principles, and as a consequence different treatment procedures are enacted.[9,10,11,12] This step, obvious enough to any practitioner with knowledge of Chinese medicine, results in a more successful outcome of treatment than a western medical diagnosis followed by some select form of Chinese medical treatment.[13] (Other researchers avoid TCM diagnosis by using Ryodoraku points (points of high conductance) however, as yet, there is no evidence to say that Ryodoraku acupuncture is as, or more, effective than adopting TCM principles.)[14]

Treatment that is not based on TCM principles could not be expected to provide as good results by virtue of the fact that researchers are intermingling two paradigms, and interchanging languages and terminology, without having first determined that the two are compatible. The term 'dysmenorrhea' may represent more than a single concept in Chinese medicine. What initially appear to be identical cases of dysmenorrhea to a western doctor, may in fact be different cases with varying manifestations when seen through the eyes of a traditional Chinese doctor. Because traditional Chinese medicine uses different criteria for diagnosis, the Chinese doctor is directed towards differential conclusions and treatment. The western diagnosis of 'dysmenorrhea' may represent, for example, dysmenorrhea due to Cold, or due to Heat, or due to Liver Qi Stasis in a traditional Chinese framework, each calling for a different treatment, but all of which appear indistinguishable to Western eyes.[15]

Thus many reports evaluating the success of pain relief with acupuncture, though appearing to be thorough research, may not be doing justice to TCM. In fact, in many papers little attempt has been made to consider the meaning and importance of Chinese terms and diagnosis. These sentiments were also iterated by Steiner[16] in 1983:

Several controlled studies on rheumatic disorders showed no demonstrable clinical effects.[17,18] However, the methods used in some of these studies did not give due credit to the general systemic effects of acupuncture. In one study, clinical observation in symmetric joint disease was based on treatment of one joint with legitimate acupuncture and the other with alternative therapy. *Use of this method, recommended by the National Institutes of Health (NIH) in 1973, is probably the result of limited understanding of theory and practice of acupuncture.*[19] [My emphasis]

Amongst the thousands of studies conducted on the management of various syndromes with acupuncture, some make no acknowledgement of reasons for point selection, some explain point selection but provide no differentiation of patients,[20] some are ignorant of the significance of stimulation variables, whilst a few, notably from China, take into consideration all of these variables.[9,12,21] A better treatment is usually the case if most of the above factors are considered. The following chapters will introduce research that confirms the importance of the careful selection of points and stimulation variables in the application of acupuncture.

Measurement of pain is a problematic task in itself, and most clinical reports of pain relief are based on subjective expressions of pain by the patient, e.g., using a scale of 0 (no pain) to 10 (the severest imaginable). People's scales would obviously vary enormously. Some experimenters have used objective indices (electroencephalogram spectral analysis) to show that pain is manageable by electroacupuncture.[85,133,134,135] Other typical types of experiments and measurement systems adopted are:

1. The mechanical pain threshold stick (spring). The tip is applied to the skin and measures grams of pressure.
2. Potassium chloride solution and electric impulses. Used commonly on rabbit ears, the pain threshold is identified by the rabbit shaking its head.

3. Potassium algometers.

4. Heat radiation pain meters developed in Japan.

5. The tail flick latency test, used with caged rats and mice. (In the tail flick latency test rats, as an example, are housed in special cages that are not long enough for their tails, which protrude from the rear of the cage. A heating lamp is applied over the tail, which begins to flick if the heat is uncomfortable. The temperature can be regulated precisely, and the tails not burned in any way. Once in this device rats are given acupuncture to see if pain is perceived differently.)

Of course, some of the problems that occur when designing research to assess acupuncture's usefulness in painful disorders are not as apparent when considering acupuncture analgesia for surgery. The style of experiments and reports mentioned above must be distinguished from the large body of experiments employing acupuncture analgesia for surgery, and it is to this task that we will now focus our attention.

Acupuncture analgesia and surgery

The beginnings of acupuncture analgesia (AA) stem from Shanghai in 1958, where it was initially used for the purpose of relieving postoperative pain and in the management of surgical dressings. Early experimentation extended its use to tonsillectomies and subsequently to more diverse and complicated surgery.[22,23,24]

After the first trials in 1958, interest spread rapidly throughout China and surgeons experimented with many different types of operation. Acupuncture analgesia operations peaked during the Cultural Revolution. In 1975, a report appearing in the Chinese Medical Journal claimed that over 600 000 operations had been performed using AA throughout China, and exhibited a 90% effectiveness.[25] This seemingly high claim of success was not unusual, and not necessarily realistic, during the Cultural Revolution. However, it is not unusual to see present day estimates of successful acupuncture analgesia having been performed on over one million operations.[22]

A significant number of operations under acupuncture analgesia were also performed on children, however a basal analgesia was incorporated for children up to age 7, as it is difficult to obtain the cooperation of young children. This aimed at keeping the child quiet, but preserving all physiological reflexes. The authors of the 1975 report claim that 2.5% sodium pentothal alone, (20 mg/kg body weight intramuscularly), is not sufficient to meet the analgesic requirements of the operations. In support they quote their earlier study[26], which compared procaine requirements for acupuncture and nonacupuncture patients all undergoing operations for inguinal hernias and using basal analgesia. The nonacupuncture patients required greater doses of procaine to continue the operation. In the study on children, the authors also found that amongst those 1062 requiring basal analgesia, 206 (19.4%)

failed. In 412 cases without basal analgesia, 62 (15%) failed. Hence, basal analgesia did not act to raise the effectiveness rate of acupuncture analgesia.

It soon became apparent that acupuncture analgesia had limitations as to the type of surgery for which it could be used, and it is currently estimated that this technique has become a preferred method in 10% to 30% of all cases.[22,23] However it should be clearly stated that in selected cases and subjects the success rate can often be over 90%.[22] (p 221)

Tables 2.1 and 2.2 indicate that AA is principally used in surgery of the head (ear, nose and throat disorders), neck and chest, and gynecological conditions. From these we can see it is particularly useful in thyroidectomy laryngectomy, internal fixation of fractures (e.g., femoral neck) and dental extraction. It is less successful for abdominal operations such as laparotomies, predominantly due to insufficient relaxation of the abdominal muscles or the discomfort of visceral traction. Under AA, sensations of pressure and traction are often retained, and muscle relaxation is poor, which restricts its use for intra-abdominal operations, unless they are simple or the abdominal wall is stretched, as for example, in caesarian sections.

From these tables and other information we know that AA is effective only to a certain degree. What factors control this level of effetiveness is the subject of a great deal of research. As the AA effectiveness varies with individuals, we can see the advantages of having at hand some useful predictors in order to make a preoperative estimation of the analgesic effect of AA. Various physiological, biological and psychological parameters have been looked at, including the radioimmunoassay (RIA) measurement of the serum levels of gastrin, endorphin, estradiol and progesterone. For example, Tang Dean claims that if serum estradiol is high in female mice then acupuncture analgesia is likely to be more successful.[27]

Chang et al claim they can test the potential AA response to acupuncture by firstly ascertaining the strength of the Qi sensation.[28] Others have reported that AA is better with Yang Xu compared with Yin Xu patients, but that this can be improved in Yin Xu subjects if their condition is treated prior to surgery.[27] Furthermore in animals AA seems to improve with maturity. The analgesic effect of acupuncture is poor in newborn mice, but in increases gradually with the development and maturation of the animal.[27] The most comprehensive studies on preoperative forecasts of the effectiveness of acupuncture anaesthesia concluded that no single physiological, biochemical or psychological index could predict with accuracy the analgesic outcome, but if these indices were combined into a mathematical formula, they provided a very accurate forecast of the effectiveness of acupuncture analgesia.[139]

This also directs our attention to the demands of AA upon patients. Do they need to be selected somewhat? It would seem that many more opt for it than are suitable, and this is an issue that future research would need to address. As we have stated, in some surgical procedures requiring deep analgesia or full muscular relaxation, AA is not sufficient.[29] AA presents a distinct advantage for older patients, however, because of the danger of

Table 2.1 Results of acupuncture analgesia in various kinds of operation (Extracted from Chinese Medical Journal 1(5): 369–374, 1975)

Regions of operation	No. of cases	Grade I	Grade II	Effective results Grade III	Total	Failures %
Head and neck	45	6	15	11	31	71.1	13
Tonsils	300	118	120	29	267	89.0	33
Chest	10	5	4	. . .	9	90.0	1
Gastrointestinal	310	83	112	48	243	78.3	67
Appendix	362	110	114	58	282	77.9	80
Other abdominal organs	134	42	48	20	108	80.6	26
Inguinal	187	71	70	33	174	93.1	13
Lumbar and sacral	26	3	10	7	20	76.9	6
Extremities	64	21	12	13	46	71.8	18
Miscellaneous	36	4	14	7	25	69.4	11
Total	1474	463	517	226	1296	81.8	268

Table 2.2 Effectiveness of acupuncture analgesia (80 000 surgical operations carried out in Shanghai hospitals to the end of May 1973 (Reproduced with permission from Needham and Lu, Celestial lancets: or history and rationale of acupuncture and moxibustion, Cambridge University Press)

Operation	Percentages Grade I	Grades I & II	Grades I, II & III	Grade IV
Craniotomy	35	71	97	3
Retinal detachment	32	73	80	20
Thyroidectomy	54	85	95	5
Total laryngectomy	54	84	93	7
Pulmonary resection	18	44	97	3
Mitral commissurotomy	32	73	94	6
Open heart surgery	12	77	87	13
Sub-total gastrectomy	17	62	96	4
Abdominal hysterectomy	34	74	85	15
Internal fixation of fractures	52	90	96	4
Caesarean section	–	–	97	3
Dental extraction	70	97	–	3
Veterinary operations	30	70	95	5

Note in both tables — Grade I: excellent analgesic effect — only slight pain; blood pressure, pulse and respiration almost normal. Grade II: good analgesia — some pain; physiological data change slightly; a local chemical analgesic may be used. Grade III: fair analgesic effect — pain, but insufficient to cease surgery or to require pethidine, although more local analgesic is given. Grade IV: poor analgesia; complete recourse to chemical anaesthesia.

anaesthetic drugs. For extended operations greater than 3 hours AA is less successful, though it has been used for up to 6 hours.[30]

In many cases because of insufficient deep analgesia, AA is supplemented by pharmacological premedication, usually small amounts of sedatives or analgesics insufficient to cause analgesia in themselves. Metoclopramide has been employed to assist AA because it has antidopamine and anticholinesterase actions. Dopamine has been shown to possess an antagonistic effect on AA, whilst increased acetylcholine levels have been correlated with successful AA.[1]

Numerous experiments have been performed in China exploring the characteristics of acupuncture induced analgesia, and shedding some light on the underlying mechanisms. Observations such as shown in Figure 2.1 were originally made on humans, but have since been repeated in studies on rats and rabbits.

Consistently, acupuncture analgesia:

1. Achieves its maximum level within 20 to 30 minutes;
2. Decreases with a half-life of 15 to 17 minutes upon removal of the needles;
3. Exhibits a slow onset and a slow wearing characteristic, suggesting that a humoral mechanism is significant.

The slow rise to a maximum level of analgesia has been confirmed by many sources,[14,31,32,33] (For a typical experiment monitoring these changes see Andersson & Holmgren.[34] All three characteristics were described in their experiment on the measurement of pain thresholds on the dental pulp of humans.)

An experiment using 306 normal persons to measure pain threshold changes by using auricular points with only manual manipulation of the needles produces some interesting and usable results.[32] Generally, the pain threshold may be raised by 100% to 200%, although depending on the individual it may be several fold or very little.[35] The principal characteristics elicited from this study are:

1. Different ear points give rise to changes in pain threshold at different parts of the body surface. For example, the Shenmen and Lung points provide the best analgesia for the chest and abdomen, whilst the Sympathetic point achieves little there. Other experimenters obtained similar results.[14]

2. The best analgesic effect occurs after 20 to 30 minutes of needling. During retention of the needle the analgesic effect remains or drops slightly. After withdrawal the analgesic effect may last for up to 2 hours whilst gradually decreasing.

3. There is no marked difference between needling one or both ears.

4. The analgesic effect is dependent upon individual characteristics such as emotions, age, and sex.

5. Manipulation of needles (by twirling) increases and maintains the pain threshold, whilst ceasing manipulation decreases the threshold.

All the characteristics so far mentioned are important considerations in the formation of a protocol for the application of acupuncture analgesia. In the West to date, such guidelines are sadly lacking and can only be a reflection of the lack of attention to this area in orthodox medical circles. Nevertheless certain conclusions regarding the advantages and disadvantages of using AA can be gleaned from our observations of clinical and experimental studies.[22,36,37,38]

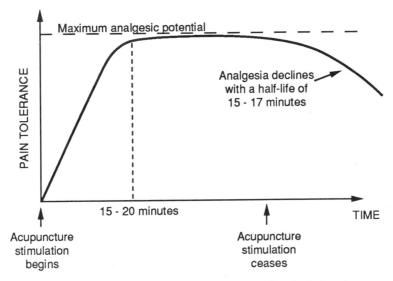

Fig. 2.1   Pattern of growth and decline of acupuncture induced analgesia (not drawn to scale).

One of the distinct advantages is that the patient is conscious and can coop-erate. For example, in thyroidectomy, trauma to the laryngeal nerve could be detected early. It is a safe procedure, free of deaths or serious complications, and there are fewer side effects postoperatively (such as nausea, vomiting, respiratory difficulty, and urine retention) than with chemical anaesthesia. Interference with physiological function is minimal, and circulation, digestion, fluid balance, and electrolyte balance remain normal. This may be particularly relevant in difficult births where no chemical agents pollute the fetus. In fact, it is apparent that acupuncture increases immunological disposition, in con-trast to the suppression of immunity subsequent to a general anaesthetic.[22] Other advantages are early mobilisation and feeding, its suitability for poor anaesthetic risks, such as the elderly, the existence in some cases of prolonged postoperative analgesia (up to 24 hrs), and the fact that it is simple, cheap, and adaptable.

On the other hand, obvious disadvantages are that the analgesia is in-complete, and there may remain sensation of touch, pressure or traction. Furthermore there is unsatisfactory muscle relaxation especially on the abdomen. AA's effectiveness is decreased markedly if the operation extends for more than three hours, although, as mentioned earlier, surgery has been performed lasting up to six hours.

Finally, some reference works are available as guides for the selection of acupuncture points for surgical analgesia, but these are basic and act only as summaries of studies already performed.[22,5] Many other acupuncture points are possible and their usage depends on the individual circumstances.

THE REGULATORY EFFECT OF ACUPUNCTURE

In 1979 the World Health Organization drew up a list of diseases that they felt were responsive to acupuncture treatment (Table 2.3).[39] This was based on clinical experience, particularly in China, and not necessarily on controlled research. However, since that time a prodigious number of clinical studies have been conducted, many of which underscore the value of acupuncture for painless disorders.

This is hardly surprising when one looks closely at what has emerged from the research efforts in AA. These investigations in analgesia have been extremely fruitful in demonstrating the widespread neurological influence of acupuncture, with all the concomitant chemical changes in neurotransmitter availability (see Chs 4 and 5). The resultant changes in the availability of parasympathetic and sympathetic neurochemical mediators will, of course, exercise a profound and pervasive physiological influence. In this section then, we will deal with the action of acupuncture in regulating bodily functions and blood chemistry, probably the most ubiquitous and significant therapeutic effect produced by needling.

The regulating effect of needling was, of course, recognised by the physicians of ancient times. We learn from Chapter 1 of the Ling Shu[132] that

Table 2.3   The WHO provisional list of diseases that lend themselves to acupuncture treatment

Upper respiratory tract	*Disorders of the mouth*
Acute sinusitis	Toothache
Acute rhinitis	Post-extraction pain
Common cold	Gingivitis
Acute tonsilitis	Acute and chronic pharyngitis
Respiratory system	*Gastrointestinal system*
Acute bronchitis	Spasms of oseophagus and cardia
Bronchial asthma	Hiccough
	Acute and chronic gastritis
Disorders of the eye	Gastric hyperacidity
Acute conjunctivitis	Chronic duodenal ulcer (pain relief)
Central retinitis	Acute duodenal ulcer (without complications)
Myopia (in children)	Acute bacillary dysentery
Cataract (without complications)	Constipation
	Diarrhoea
	Paralytic ileus

Neurological and musculoskeletal disorders	
Headache	Nocturnal enuresis
Migraine	Intercostal neuralgia
Trigeminal neuralgia	Cervicobrachial syndrome
Facial palsy (early stage)	'Frozen shoulder'
Pareses following a stroke	'Tennis elbow'
Peripheral neuropathies	Sciatica
Sequelae of poliomyelitis (early stage)	Low back pain
Meniere's disease	Osteoarthritis
Neurogenic bladder dysfunction	

acupuncture can keep the channels open, regulate the Blood and Qi and balance Excess and Deficiency conditions.

The spectrum of functional changes brought about by acupuncture may be as widespread as:

- Controlling the movement of substances within the body, for example, peristaltic activity in the digestive process, or smooth muscle influence in the control of urination and childbirth;
- Altering hemodynamics, such as blood pressure, cardiac output and microcirculation;
- Promoting antishock mechanisms in the body, (needling promotes survival of the subject).

The modification of body or blood chemistry due to needling may also be wide ranging and evidenced by:

- Production of enzymes and hormones;
- Changes in cellular and humoral immunity;
- Alterations of blood cell counts, for example, white blood cells and platelets.

In the following we will explore the nature of each of these functional or chemical changes, with the exception of the acupuncture influences on immunity, which have been allocated a later section. It is important to note that by no means should this be interpreted as a comprehensive and all inclusive review of the regulating effect of acupuncture. It is presented to exemplify the extent and direction of influence that acupuncture is able to exert.

Functional changes

Acupuncture has been shown to be effective in the attenuation of exercise induced asthma.[40] Forced expiratory flow, forced vital capacity and peak expiratory flow rate were measured throughout acupuncture and after treadmill exercise, with the result that real acupuncture provided better protection against exercise induced asthma than did sham acupuncture.

Acupuncture was also effective in reversing bronchospasm from methacholine inhalation[41] athough isoproterenol was more effective.[42] Acupuncture generally improves bronchoconstriction and pulmonary function during clinical attacks of asthma.[43,44] In a more recent study, the subjective reporting of breathlessness in patients with chronic obstructive pulmonary disease was improved, although objective indices of lung function remained unchanged.[21] It is interesting to note that, published in December 1986, this paper was the first to appear in the *Lancet* where traditional Chinese diagnosis has been respected.

In an earlier paper, Tashkin and Bresler demonstrated a statistically significant improvement in lung function in acute experimentally induced bronchospasm.[42] However, in subsequent research they contradicted their own earlier studies to find that acupuncture failed to reveal a significant effect on symptoms, medication use, or lung funtion measurements.[20] In both experiments a standard set of acupuncture loci were used and no TCM diagnosis of patients was attempted, problems highlighted earlier as being detrimental to any genuine study.

Polish studies in 1984 furnished optimistic results that patients with chronic bronchitis who had a long term reliance on oral or intramuscular corticosteroids also had a good chance of eliminating their dependence with extended acupuncture treatment (63.8% of patients succeeded).[45] Acupuncture therefore, it was claimed, exerts a favourable influence on the stimulation of natural steroids. The amounts of plasma histamine, acetylcholine and adrenalin are also all relevant factors in asthma, and we shall see in Chapters 4 and 5 just how obvious a role they play in acupuncture.

In obstetrics acupuncture has been employed, not only to relieve the pain of labour and delivery,[46,47,48] but also to induce labour.[49,50,51] This has included studies on initiating contractions prior to the rupture of the membranes, and prior to the patient experiencing any labour pains.[52] Other investigators, commenting on their findings, noted that under acupuncture 'the relation between the force of contraction and the degree of dilation of the cervix differed from that in oxytocin induced and spontaneous labour' (p 337).[53] Even more dramatic results have come from studies in China. In Guizhou auricular acupuncture was successfully used for dilatation of the cervical os, where, because of its tightness, artificial abortion and diagnostic curettage had proved impossible.[54] In Yunnan, using volunteers who had applied for abortion or induction of labour, it was found that needling Hegu (Co 4) and Sanyinjiao (Sp 6) could initiate uterine contractions at any stage of pregnancy, including the first term.[55] In West Germany, auricular acupuncture was used in women with infertility, 15 associated with oligomenorrhea and 12 associated with luteal body insufficiency. In both groups the subsequent incidence of pregnancy was comparable to that achieved by drug therapy.[142]

The Shanghai Medical College acupuncture textbook[5] summarises a large number of experiments and recent experience in China on the functional changes in the digestive system induced by acupuncture. Although original Chinese sources have been difficult to obtain it is worthwhile repeating here the synthesis of observations presented in this college textbook:

After needling Zusanli (St 36) on a normal subject, the amplitude and frequency of peristalsis in the stomach increased, the tension was raised, the stomach emptying time was shortened and the period of contraction of the stomach lengthened.
Needling Zusanli (St 36) and related points on patients with gastric ulcers will, in most cases, cause an increase in peristalsis, open the pyloris and accelerate the emptying time of the stomach. In research carried out by Xian No. 1 Hospital it was found that needling certain points caused a retardation of stomach functions, while needling other points can cause an acceleration of the gastric functions.
The effects of acupuncture on patients with intestinal tract disorders were even more

pronounced. For instance, clinical studies in Guangdong province, among patients with intestinal obstruction due to roundworm, or with partial intestinal obstruction, showed that after stimulation of Sifeng (M-UE 9), there was an expansion of certain segments of the intestinal tract, relief from intestinal cramps, and generally an acceleration of peristalsis as well as the speed with which the intestines were emptied. (p 529)

Of greater interest is the fact that the Shanghai College determined that if gastric function was hypoactive, then gastrointestinal activity would be stimulated, whilst it would be inhibited if gastric function were hyperactive. Furthermore, levels of free stomach acids, pepsin and gastric lipase could all be returned to normal. This has been supported more recently by studies conducted in Nigeria on patients with duodenal ulcers.[56] The output of gastric acid in the duodenal ulcer group was markedly reduced, and the authors agreed that the relief of pain in chronic duodenal ulcer patients was probably attributable to the therapeutic inhibition of gastric hyperacidity in the patients. They go on to say that 'though pain relief has been previously demonstrated in response to acupuncture, the results of this investigation have gone further to show that acupuncture achieves symptomatic relief through therapeutic gastric depression in duodenal ulcer patients'. (p 356)

The Chinese claim similar changes have been confirmed in the alteration of frequency and amplitude of peristalsis in the colon and contraction of the sphincter of Oddi (gall bladder).[5] But as the bulk of the original research is difficult to obtain, it is impossible to verify the levels of control and standards of data collection exercised in these experiments. It is appropriate to mention that at that time in China, control groups were rarely used in clinical trials. However, more recent and controlled work has been carried out which endorses the earlier findings of the Chinese. Reporting in the *American Journal of Surgery*, Matsumoto and Hayes found that gastrointestinal motility could be improved after complete bilateral truncal vagotomy in rabbits.[57] Electroacupuncture succeeded, in comparison with the control group, in increasing bowel motility postoperatively. Similarly, needling Zusanli (St 36) during fibroptic gastroscopy was found to be helpful in relieving upper gastrointestinal tract spasm, despite the failure of premedication.[58,136] The acupuncture point Neiguan (Per 6) has also been reported in the *British Medical Journal* as providing a significant reduction in perioperative nausea and vomiting.[3]

Altering haemodynamics

Needling has been shown to improve many hemodynamic disturbances. Omura demonstrated that acupuncture produced prolonged augmentation of microcirculation in peripheral tissue and the brain.[59] Improved circulation would counteract local muscle spasm, vasospasm and ischemia. The effects of needling on nail microcirculation, as a reflection of blood flow velocity, was also confirmed by Chen et al in Beijing.[60] Furthermore, they claim the variation in microcirculation and skin temperature local to the point of needle insertion is a reflection of the specific needle technique used.

Cardiovascular function is specifically moderated by acupuncture.[61] Do Chil Lee and colleagues confirmed that acupuncture at Renzhong (Du 26) on dogs produced sympathomimetic effects on the cardiovascular system, such as increased cardiac output and heart rate, and that these effects are inhibited by propranolol.[62,63,64,65] In contrast, acupuncture at Zusanli (St 36) was shown to produce parasympathomimetic effects on the cardiovascular system, such as decreased blood pressure and slower heart rate, which were inhibited by atropine. The effects of acupuncture in decreasing hypertension have also been studied elsewhere in human and animal subjects.[66,67,68]

Whilst acupuncture at Yangxi (Co 5) was effective in correcting pulsus alternans and sinus arrhythmia in dogs[65], stimulation of the Renying point (St 9) was successful enough to reverse experimentally induced cardiac arrest. Cardiac arrest followed the administration of 1% halothane in 6% oxygen, 10% carbon dioxide and 83% nitrogen for approximately 20 minutes. Dogs exposed to these percentages of inhaled gases develop hypotension and cardiac arrest followed by death.[69] In two dogs that developed cardiac arrest, acupuncture at Renying (St 9) returned cardiovascular function to normal. Two other dogs who did not receive acupuncture died.

Also experimenting with dogs, Li Peng, Sun Fengyen and Zhang Anzhong in the Shanghai First Medical College discovered that needling Zusanli (St 36) produced a significant decrease in blood pressure which was naloxone reversible and hence calculated to be mediated by endogenous opioids released under acupuncture.[70] This was also confirmed by the ineffectiveness of acupuncture in reducing blood pressure in anaesthetised dogs, an observation made in China and the USA.[65] Importantly, the workers of Shanghai First Medical College demonstrated the presence of opiate receptors in blood vessels, and this provides direct evidence for the peptidergic peripheral mediation of blood pressure. Other authors had also previously speculated or identified the existence of peripheral receptors that respond to opioids in the blood circulation.[71,72,73,74]

Researchers have also shown that ischaemic damage due to blockage of coronary supply may be minimised with electrical needling at Neiguan (Per 6).[75,76,77,78] Others still have monitored changes in electrocardiograms and cardiac echos.[79,80,81,82]

The *anti—shock effect of needling* is another important characteristic which is observed most easily in human and animal subjects that are under acupuncture analgesia. As mentioned earlier, despite the psychological and physical stresses of surgery, normal physiological functions such as blood pressure and respiration are usually maintained. The anti-shock mechanism of acupuncture is considered to operate via the activation of the sympathetic and parasympathetic nervous systems. It exerts a regulatory function in alleviating bronchospasm, improving respiratory function, reducing pulmonary stasis, and decreasing hemodynamic disorder.

In experiments performed by Mu Jian at Nanjing Medical College, it was observed that allergic shock induced by penicillin or serum anaphylaxis could be successfully controlled with the help of acupuncture. Various levels of control were designed in this experiment, which reduced the death rate of mice to one third that of the major control group, whilst the symptoms of shock were markedly alleviated.[83] More importantly, in subsequent experiments Mu Jian found this needling effect was antagonised by phentolamine (alpha-adrenergic receptor antagonist), and propanolol (beta 2-adrenergic blocker), but remained constant after injection of practolol (beta 1-adrenergic blocker).[84] The implication is that alpha and beta 2-adrenergic receptors are involved in the electroacupuncture anti-allergic effect. Furthermore, naloxone injections or previous exhaustion of pituitary endorphins did not affect the outcome, suggesting that different mechanisms underly the anti-shock, as opposed to analgesic, effect of acupuncture. Electroconvulsive shock also responds favourably to acupuncture.[85]

In another study 18 dogs had their blood pressure lowered from approximately 147 mmHg to 90 mmHg by artificial bleeding. Each dog lost 15 ml of blood per kilogram of body weight in a short time. Half the dogs were then given electroacupuncture and the others nothing. Those without acupuncture suffered low cardiac output, high peripheral resistance, and decreased visceral circulation.[32]

Biochemical alterations

Acupuncture may also produce a definite regulatory effect on body and blood chemistry. This response can occur immediately, although Omura claims that the alterations of blood chemistry begin only after 4 hours and reach a peak between seven and 24 hours in most cases.[59]

It has already been mentioned that studies conducted in the Shanghai College of TCM, and summarised in the Shanghai text, demonstrated that needling (St 36, Co 4, Sp 6) may restore levels of stomach acidity, free stomach acids, pepsin, and gastric lipase.[5] Release of pancreatic juice and bile were also shown to occur with the needling of certain points.

More recently, Ionescu-Tirgoviste and Mincu performed interesting studies on blood sugar levels in patients with diabetes.[86] Needling Sanyinjiao (Sp 6) in non-insulin dependent diabetics resulted in decreased glycemia 2 to 4 hours after stimulation in 94% of the patients needled. Stimulating the same point in insulin dependent diabetic patients produced an increase in glycemia in a similar time span for 87% of patients. This action was specific to Sanyinjiao (Sp 6), as using other points could not mimic its effects. Once again acupuncture exhibited a physiologically normalising effect, in this case on the pancreas. However, Polish researchers found that human plasma insulin levels decreased after acupuncture in healthy subjects, and that this may be related to alpha-adrenergic activity.[87]

Studies in Japan on rabbits demonstrated that puncturing Zusanli (St 36) affected citrate metabolism in the liver so as to increase the production of glucose, and reduce that of ketone body, free cholesterol and free fatty acid, however it exerted no effect on glucose metabolism in the liver.[88] When placed under stressful conditions (such as heat, cold and immobilisation) both citrate and glucose metabolism were affected, but this could be moderated by puncturing Zusanli (St 36).

As we shall see in Chapter 4, acupuncture significantly affects the pituitary as this is a major site for the release of endogenous opioid peptides. This in turn has repercussions on other endocrine glands, such as the adrenal cortex. For example, it has been reported that serum and urine content of 17-OHCS (hydroxycorticosteroid) and 17-ketosteriod are altered with acupuncture, although the experimental conditions are unclear from the report.[5,89] Wen and colleagues demonstrated positive alterations of adrenocorticotropic hormone (ACTH) levels when treating drug addicts with true acupuncture.[90,91] Adrenal production of corticosterone and cortisol was also enhanced in rabbits by needling at Zusanli (St 36) as opposed to sham acupuncture at a non-locus.[92]

Across to the other side of the Pacific, in the USA, it was demonstrated that acupuncture could induce decreases in the blood concentrations of triglycerides, cholesterol and phospholipids in 206 patients with essential hypertension, although the decrease in cholesterol was less significant.[59] The average changes are cited in Table 2.4.

Table 2.4   Average changes in triglyceride, cholesterol and phospholipid levels under acupuncture (Reprinted with permission from Acupuncture and Electrotherapeutics Research, Vol. 1, Omura, Y., Pathophysiology of acupuncture treatment: effect of acupuncture on cardiovascular and nervous systems, Copyright 1975, Pergamon Press PLC)

	Normal range (mg/100ml)	Before acup. (mg/100ml)	8 hrs after (mg/100ml)	1 wk after (mg/100ml)
Triglycerides	50–100	235	107	150
Cholesterol	150–300	314	285	290
Phospholipid	150–300	339	197	200

Of course there are many other aspects of the acupuncture related changes in blood chemistry that ought to be considered. Cellular (white blood cell and sensitised lymphocyte) and humoral immune abilities are capable of being raised with acupuncture. Although both will be addressed more thoroughly when discussing the immunity enhancing functions of acupuncture, it is worthwhile drawing attention to some aspects of white blood cell count (WBCC) alterations under acupuncture. Most importantly it has been observed that different manipulations will induce different results, as shown in Figure 2.2. The new white blood cell count may persist for 1 to 3 hours after needling.[32]

Secondly, Professor Mu Jian of Nanjing Medical College reports that different effects are produced by needling different points. For example, Yamen

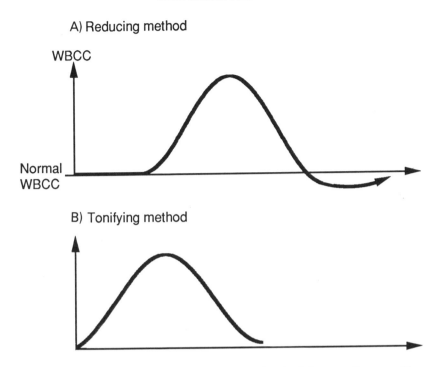

A) Reducing method

WBCC

Normal
WBCC

B) Tonifying method

The new white blood cell counts may persist 1 - 3 hours after needling

Fig. 2.2 Different needle manipulations result in different patterns of variation of white blood cell counts (WBCC).

(Du 15) and Huagai (Ren 20) may lead to an increased WBCC and increased haemopoietic function of bone marrow. Naohu (Du 17), on the other hand, causes a decrease in WBCC and an increase in lymphocytes.[32]

The importance of these last two points is that they illustrate the significance of precise point location and manipulation, a case that is argued more fully below. These results exist in stark contrast to one report that claims simple penetration of the skin will stimulate immune factors equally well. Brown, Ulett and Stern state there is no difference between the stimulation of a real point or a nonpoint on white blood cell count.[93] However, it is possible that the points selected were inappropriate to increase white cell count, and any responses at those acupuncture points was similar to stress responses of needling elsewhere.

Acupuncture can temporarily raise white blood cell count in patients with weak resistance and poor immune functions. For example, 25 cases of leukopenia resulting from radio- and chemotherapy were treated by needling Zuxanli (St 36), Sanyinjiao (Sp 6), Xuanzhong (GB 39), Xuehai (Sp 10), and Geshu (Bl 17) as the main points. On average the white blood cell count was elevated by 5128/mm^3 after a period of treatment.[32] Similarly, acupuncture assisted recovery of depressed total leukocyte count in gamma irradiated mice.[94] In another experiment on X-irradiated rats plasma leukocytes, lymphocytes and neutrocytes were all elevated after electroacupuncture compared with the control groups.[95]

Normal healthy persons receiving acupuncture generally have their white blood cell counts raised, or transiently lowered then raised. The latter pattern of biphasic change seems quite common and is confirmed by several researchers.[59,96] In animal studies 15 normal rabbits were needled at Zusanli (St 36) with the result that prior to needling the white blood cell count was 13 598/mm^3, 30 minutes after it was 12 364, 3 hours after it was 22 600 (166% of preacupuncture value), and 7.5 hours after it returned to normal.[32]

Needling also has a regulatory effect on blood platelet and other coagulent factors. Clinical reports claim that acupuncture gives a definite therapeutic effect on primary thrombocytopenic purpura and other haemorrhagic diseases. Blood coagulation took much less time in patients 30 minutes after needling and the prothrombin index was increased by 13.5%.[32] Chu reported that while acupuncture treatments tended to increase the blood sedimentation rate initially, after the eighth treatment this rate returned to within normal limits. The number of erythrocytes usually increased after the first treatment.[97]

As we have seen above, the ability to regulate physiological functions and body chemistry gives credibility to the potential of acupuncture to act as a preventive and curative form of therapy. The regulating properties of acupuncture are ubiquitous in that they may be observed to a certain degree in many of the bodily systems; digestive, urinary, circulatory, cardiovascular, nervous, and endocrine. The many neurochemical responses to acupuncture provide a sound physiological basis for the clinical observations reported in this section. Once we define and monitor sympathetic and parasympathetic neurological changes, it is a straight forward step to acknowledge acupuncture's influence on endocrine systems, enzyme responses and even immunological behaviour. To this latter category we will now direct our attention.

RAISING THE IMMUNITY OF THE BODY

The classics emphasise that acupuncture and moxibustion 'strengthen bodily resistance'. What does this mean in biological terms? Clinical surveys illustrate, for example, that viral, bacterial and protozoal infections may be effectively treated with acupuncture.[98] In order to understand this in the western biomedical framework we need to inspect more closely the possible range of changes in the immune system that are brought about by acupuncture. The following four areas warrant review:

1. Changes brought about in the cellular immune ability of the body — white blood cells, sensitised T-lymphocytes and their phagocytic activity;
2. Changes brought about in the humoral immune ability — production of antibodies (immunoglobulins) by B-lymphocytes;

3. Changes brought about in the reticuloendothelial system (mobile and fixed tissue macrophages (in liver, lymph nodes, spleen, bone marrow) and phagocytic activity;
4. The anti-allergic effect of needling (suppressing hypersensitivity).

Cellular immune ability

Because of the relationship between immune responses and stress, this is an area of significant scepticism in acupuncture research. Some authors claim that simple penetration of the skin, as a stress response, will stimulate immune factors equally well, and state there is little difference between needling real acupuncture points and nonpoints.[99,100]

When an area of the skin anywhere on the body is stimulated, the immune/ inflammatory system is mobilised. This reaction to acupuncture may involve histamine, bradykinin, cyclic AMP, serotonin, prostaglandins, and a variety of substances yet to be discovered. (p 82)[99]

Other investigators maintain that the immune system is definitely stimulated by acupuncture and this can be contrasted with stress responses. For example, Min highlights the difference by restraining his control group of mice (rather than needling at non-sites) and claims that electroacupuncture at Dazhui (Du 14) enhances phagocytic activity of the reticuloendothelial system, unlike the negligible manifestation of stress due to restraint.[101] On the other hand, although also using one control group without acupuncture, Chu and Affronti assessed the efficacy of needling Zusanli (St 36) in comparison with Dazhui (Du 14) on raising the antibody titre in rabbits.[102] In this case the animals needled with one point double up as a control group for those animals needled with the other point. Interestingly Chu and Affronti discovered there was no change of plasma antibodies when needling Dazhui (Du 14), but that the antibody titre did increase by two — to eightfold when Zusanli (St 36) or Quchi (Co 11) were needled. This certainly swings support behind the Chinese claim that points exhibit *specific* functions. One reason for the appearance of contradictory findings may well rest on the fact that more precise point selection is required during experimentation.

There have been considerable experimental observations regarding the influence of needling on cellular immunity. Some indicate the promotion of lymphocyte activity and increases in lymphocyte blastogenesis rate after needling.[32] Ding, Roath and Lewith found that circulating lymphocytes increased after needling Zusanli (St 36) but only lasted a few hours.[103] In China, experiments on asthmatic children demonstrated a definite enhancement of all immunological function, particularly if acupuncture was supported by substantial propagation of needling sensation along the channel.[104] Other studies in China at Henan Medical College ascertained via E-rosette tests and assays of lymphocyte transformation that electroacupuncture boosted cell mediated immunity.[137]

Humoral immune ability

Acupuncture may significantly raise the titres of humoral immune factors such as bacteriolysin (antibody that breaks down bacteria); complement (series of substances with actions on antigen and antibody reaction); agglutinin (immunoglobulin that causes agglutination and facilitates phagocytosis); opsonin (antibody that renders bacteria and other cells susceptible to phagocytosis); and precipitin (antibody that causes antigens to aggregate and precipitate).

Experiments consistently show that introducing an antigen, for example, by way of vaccines, and subsequently performing acupuncture will markedly increase antibody titres, in contrast with control groups who have had vaccine introduced but no acupuncture.[32,102]

In one report various antigens were injected into rats, pigs and rabbits.[32] Hegu (Co 4) and Xuanzhong (GB 39) were needled immediately after inocculation. The antibody titre rose quickly and reached a higher peak, which persisted compared to the control group. (In some cases this peak persisted for 30 to 50 days.) Other experiments show that if a vaccine is injected and followed by acupuncture, one needs only a fraction (for example, one seventh) of the vaccine to attain the same antibody titre in the immunised patient.[138] This has obvious implications for anywhere there is a shortage of vaccine (such as developing nations). In separate studies in China it was discovered that electroacupuncture helped to recover the concentrations of alpha-, beta- and gamma-globulin in X-irradiated rats.[95]

Reticuloendothelial system

Studies exist that illustrate needling may also increase phagocytic activity of the reticuloendothelial system. Most experiments have been concerned with rabbits and mice. At the Research Institute of TCM (Jiangsu) ink particles were administered to 36 rabbits (others have used carbon) to determine the rate at which the foreign particles are engulfed (phagocytic activity) by the liver.[105] The rabbits were divided into three groups with the principal control group being restrained but not needled. The rabbits were killed and their livers inspected for phagocytic activity 1, 6, 15, and 20 days after cessation of needling. On the 1st day after acupuncture, phagocytic activity was 7.1% higher than that of the control group. However, on the 6th day this increased to 49% and finally on the 10th day it was 63% higher than the control group.

Anti-allergic effect of needling

The anti-allergic effect of needling refers to the ability of acupuncture to suppress hypersensitivity of the organism. As the following two examples illustrate, it is clear that acupuncture has anti-allergic functions:

1. Mu Jian made mice allergic with cow serum, and the allergic dose was used to cause, under normal conditions, a death rate of approximately 75%. The application of electroacupuncture to Renzhong (Du 26) and Chengjiang (Ren 24) at the time of allergy could lower the death rate to 26.6%.[106]

2. Guinea pigs were made to have experimental allergic encephalitis by the injection of a liquid preparation in the brainstem. They were subsequently needled at Zhishi (Bl 52) daily resulting in a slowing down of the allergic encephalitis with an alleviation of symptoms and signs.[102] (Note that locus Zhishi (Bl 52) has in the past been claimed to instigate the release of endogenous ACTH).[107]

In an experiment report in the *American Journal of Chinese Medicine*, Lau et al treated 22 subjects with allergic rhinitis. 19 patients voiced a significant decrease in the subjective rating of symptoms and this correlated with a decrease in absolute numbers of blood eosinophils, and the percentage of nasal eosinophils. Furthermore, immunoglobulin IgE levels decreased in 64% of subjects after a course of six treatments.[108] Similar falls in IgE levels were determined in asthmatic children (the release of histamine elicits the production of IgE) and this coincided with rises in plasma cAMP and T-lymphocyte immunological function.[104]

As a final note it may be worthwhile registering the observation that in cases where acupuncture analgesia is adopted postoperative infection is rarely seen, and healing of the incision is faster than otherwise. This is may be related to the stimulation of the immune system by needling. As quoted from the Shanghai College textbook[5]:

Acupuncture ... may strengthen the ability of cells to repair themselves and produce scar tissue. It was discovered after needling St 36 and St 41 on cats with ulcers of the caecum, that the alkaline phosphate reactions in the production of new epidermal skin cells occurred stronger and sooner. This is helpful in the generation and return of function of the tissues. (p 534)

THE SEDATIVE AND PSYCHOLOGICAL EFFECT OF NEEDLING

It is commonly known to practitioners that acupuncture is capable of treating anxiety, neurosis, mania, depression, insomnia, and a whole range of psychological and emotional disorders. Without overlooking the need to address social and environmental issues, acupuncture, like drug therapy, has significant short- and long-term solutions to offer.

Following from Dr Wen's observations in the early 1970s on the treatment of drug addicts with acupuncture[90,91], Shaub and Haq explored the possibility of using similar electroacupuncture therapy in psychiatric disorders.[109] 40 patients were selected who had all been on drug therapy for more than 6 months, suffered chronic anxiety, depression, or hysteria, but were not exhibiting schizophrenic symptoms. In 1976 their study concluded that electroacupuncture was useful in the treatment of these neurotic symptoms, and that it was cheaper and safer than other methods of treatment currently in use, including electroconvulsive therapy.

As if to fill the gap, 10 years later, in 1986, the Chinese produced a report of a study on 500 schizophrenic patients.[110] The patients were classified according to traditional Chinese medicine prior to receiving acupuncture. Shi Zhengxiu and Tan Meizhun claimed that 55% of the patients (275) were cured, but that follow up studies demonstrated about one third of these suffered relapses in the following 2 years. A significant number of remaining patients not classified as cured still showed considerable improvement in symptoms. The most important correlation with the success of acupuncture was the duration of the disease. The success rate dropped by over one third for patients who had suffered for 10 years or more.

Others have been less impressed with acupuncture therapy for mental disturbances. In Germany, Fischer et al were disappointed with their results for depressive psychosis, and observed only slightly better successes in cases of nervousness and insomnia.[111] However, they made no attempt at a differential diagnosis of patients in Chinese terms, which augered badly for their experimental outcome.

Still in Europe, an Italian group at Padua University used auricular acupuncture and determined it to be effective in reducing hallucinations and visual, auditory and somatosensitive disturbances that followed ketamine anaesthesia.[112] In a subsequent study, the Italians also explored mechanisms behind this antipsychotic function of acupuncture.[113] The intravenous anaesthetic ketamine produces various psychic disturbances when the patient regains consciousness, including hallucinations, psychomotor agitation and psychoataxia. The Italians found that acupuncture, through its strengthening of the serotonergic system, inhibits the hyperactivity of the dopaminergic system, a consequence of the anaesthesia, and thereby controls the postoperative psychotic responses.

Researchers have hypothesised that the calming, tranquillising effect of acupuncture is a response to the regulation of the metabolism of serotonin, noradrenalin, adenosine cyclophosphate, acetylcholine and other neurotransmitters, as well as its alteration of brain potentials.[110]

Conclusion

There is significant evidence that acupuncture has a pronounced analgesic effect on pain, a desirable regulatory action on the functions of organs, is supportive of the body's immunity, and possesses a calming psychological effect. All these actions exist simultaneously, and reinforce and complement each other. The total therapeutic result of acupuncture is an amalgamation of these actions, working in a direction that favours and promotes the life of the organism. With the gradual growth of information, not only is there an improvement in the understanding of the workings of the therapy, but also an expanded vision of possibilities for the future application of acupuncture.

RELATIONSHIP BETWEEN ELECTROSTIMULATION PARAMETERS AND THERAPEUTIC RESULTS

For all our discussions of the physiological effects of acupuncture, so far little has been mentioned of the influence of stimulation parameters on the therapeutic outcome. Yet it is clear factors such as electrostimulation intensity or frequency are likely to have an effect on the physiological result of needling.

Stimulation intensity

As an example, animal experiments in China have shown that for a fixed frequency (1 to 1.5 Hz) the best current intensity in order to obtain analgesia is approximately 50% of the maximum intensity the animals can tolerate[32], although under some experimental conditions (with different electric parameters) the stimulation intensity may be raised for a strong analgesic result to the maximum tolerable level.[114] (Of course, a gradual increase in intensity during acupuncture anaesthesia will improve the therapeutic result by avoiding adaptation to that level of intensity.)

Cao Xiaoding and colleagues experimented with rabbits using two intensities of electroacupuncture.[115] They found that for 20 minutes of electroacupuncture with their regular parameters (3 Hz, 4 volts, 12 mA, 0.5 ms) there was a fall in plasma noradrenalin and cyclic AMP, and that the analgesia so induced could be partly reversed by naloxone. However, if the intensity alone were increased to 25 mA (causing the rabbits to struggle hard), plasma noradrenalin, cyclic AMP and cortisol all increased markedly, and the analgesia was no longer naloxone reversible. The high cortisol level may imply the existence of stress analgesia under the strong intensity electroacupuncture.[116] Cao's results replicated the findings of Zhang Anzhong[117] 3 years previously, although Zhang had used slightly different electrical parameters. Of greater interest here is that the analgesia levels remained basically the same, implying that it is not necessary to turn up the intensity to achieve greater analgesia. However, if it were the intention to engage different neurohumoral pathways, attention to stimulation intensity may be warranted.

Whether the mechanism of electroacupuncture is similar to that of manual acupuncture is still in debate, although researchers in Italy presented interesting work on the different releasing effects of traditional manual acupuncture and electroacupuncture.[118] Under their particular experimental conditions, the Italians observed that a simultaneous increase occurred in the plasma concentration of beta-lipotropin, beta-endorphin and ACTH under electroacupuncture, whilst only very transient (5 minute) increases occurred in beta-lipotropin and beta-endorphin levels under manual stimulation.

Stimulation frequency

Clinical studies in China, Canada and Sweden on animals and human subjects have separately confirmed that, by switching frequencies of electroacupuncture, we may be able to activate different neuropeptides.[119,120] Summarising several studies in Canada, Pomeranz concluded that at low frequencies of electrostimulation (two to six Hertz) the analgesia induced was mediated by endorphins[121,122], whilst at higher frequencies such as 200 Hz, the analgesia was mediated by serotonin,[123,124,125] although dynorphins are also found to be an active component of analgesia at the higher frequencies.[126] Han and Terenius observed that low frequency electroacupuncture raises beta-endorphin levels in the cerebrospinal fluid.[71]

The management of addictions with electrostimulation also provides some confirmation for the physiological differences brought about by variable stimulation frequencies. Experimenting in acupuncture anaesthesia in Hong Kong, Meg Patterson's curiosity was aroused to explore further the possibility of the management of drug addiction with electroacupuncture. Her conclusions reported in 1975[127] and 1987[128] were that narcotic and sedative addictions responded best to the frequency range of 75 to 300 Hz; amphetamines in the ranges of 1 to 2 kHz; and cigarettes (nicotine) in the range of 5 to 10 Hz. Alcoholics also responded to the lower ranges. Meg Patterson also observed that depressive patients responded to higher frequencies and tense patients to lower frequencies.

In summation, these findings on the distinct physiological responses to the frequency of electroacupuncture stimulation highlight the importance of awareness of this factor in clinical studies, and they may also provide some insight as to why different needle manipulation techniques are claimed to induce different results in patients.

In fact, recent animal studies by Chen Zhenqiu and colleagues produced interesting results on the different effects of classical reinforcing and reducing manipulations. The reducing method prolonged the latency of the tail flick response, and the reinforcing method elevated skin temperatures significantly more than the reducing method.[129]

Relative specificity of acupuncture points

The relative specificity of acupuncture points is assumed to be closely related to the distribution of nerves. Li and colleagues in Beijing illustrated that needling Huantiao (GB 30) (ipsilaterally) and Renzhong (Du 26) inhibited nociceptive responses in rats, more so than needling Tinghui (GB 2) and Huantiao (GB 30) (contralaterally).[130] Of greater interest was the work of Takeshige in Japan, who demonstrated that acupuncture points produced an analgesia of a different nature compared with non-acupuncture points.[131] His research provides a strong argument for the distinctive nature of acupuncture treatments, a case which is taken up in greater detail in the context of the placebo effect in Chapter 4.

Number and frequency of treatments

Although little research has been specifically focused on this area, studies on the physiological effects of acupuncture indicate that an increased number of treatments lead to an increase in benefit up to a point. Tang Dean reports on the use of moxa on Bauhui (Du 20) and Shenshu (Bl 23) on rabbits daily for 9 days. The white blood cell count, serum complement level and immunoglobulins (IgG) all increased daily until the 5th day at which time they attained a peak and then returned to normal.[27] Studies by Eriksson and colleagues in Sweden report that the long-term analgesic results in the management of chronic pain are a measure of the success of cumulative acupuncture treatments.[140]

REFERENCES

1. Xu Z B, Pan Y Y, Xu S F, Mo W Y, Cao X D, He L F 1983 Synergism between metoclopramide and electroacupuncture analgesia. Acupuncture and Electrotherapeutics Research 8(3/4): 283–288
2. Han D Y, Ai C T, Liu A L, Li S W, Zhang X S 1981 Spleen point in face acupuncture used in fibrogastroscopy; an observation of fifty cases. Journal of Traditional Chinese Medicine 1(2): 144–145
3. Dundee J W, Chestnut W N, Ghally R G, Lynas A G A 1986 Traditional Chinese acupuncture: a potentially useful antiemetic? British Medical Journal 293 (Sept): 583–584
4. Xia Y Q, Zhang D, Yang C X, Xu H L, Li Y, Ma L T 1986 An approach to the effect on tumors of acupuncture in combination with radiotherapy or chemotherapy. Journal of Traditional Chinese Medicine 6(1): 23–26
5. Shanghai College of Traditional Chinese Medicine 1983 Acupuncture: a comprehensive text. O,Connor J, Bensky D (trans). Eastland Press, Chicago
6. National Health and Medical Research Council 1988 Report of the working party on acupuncture. Australian Government Publishing Service, Canberra
7. Basbaum A I, Fields H L 1984 Endogenous pain control systems: brainstem spinal pathways and endorphin circuitry. Annual Review of Neuroscience 7: 309–338
8. Watkins L R, Mayer D J 1982 Organisation of endogenous opiate and non-opiate pain control systems. Science 216: 1185–1192
9. Chen Z L, Zhou X F 1984 Effect of acupuncture in 300 cases of acute lumbar sprain. Journal of Traditional Chinese Medicine 4(2): 93
10. Sun L Y 1987 Efficacy of acupuncture in treating 100 cases of lumbago. Journal of Traditional Chinese Medicine 7(1): 23–24
11. Zhao R J 1987 39 cases of morning sickness treated with acupuncture. Journal of Traditional Chinese Medicine 7(1): 25–26
12. Jiang Y G, Mu J S, Zhang X Y, Bai Q L 1984 Clinical observation of acupuncture treatment of 106 cases of trunk sciatica. Journal of Traditional Chinese Medicine 4(3): 183–185
13. Mendelson G, Selwood T S, Kranz H, Loh T S, Kidson M A, Scott D S 1983 Acupuncture treatment of chronic back pain: a double-blind placebo-controlled trial. American Journal of Medicine 74: 49–55
14. Hyodo M, Kitade T 1976 The effects of stimulation of ear acupuncture loci on the body's pain threshold. In: Hyodo M 1977 Recent advances in acupuncture treatment (Part II). Osaka Medical College (Publ), Osaka
15. Wang X M 1987 Observations of the therapeutic effects of acupuncture and moxibustion in 100 cases of dysmenorrhea. Journal of Traditional Chinese Medicine 7(1): 15–17
16. Steiner R P 1983 Acupuncture — cultural perspectives. Postgraduate Medicine 74(4): 60–67

17. Moore M E, Berk S N 1976 Acupuncture for chronic shoulder pain: an experimental study with attention to the role of the placebo and hypnotic susceptibilty. Annals of Internal Medicine 84(4): 381–384
18. Gaw A C, Chang L W, Shaw L C 1975 Efficacy of acupuncture on osteoarthritic pain: a controlled double-blind study. New England Journal of Medicine 293(8): 375–378
19. Workshop on the use of acupuncture in the rheumatic diseases. National Institutes of Health, Bethesda, Maryland, Sep 17–18, 1973. Summary of proceedings. Arthritis and Rheumatism 17(6): 939–943, 1974
20. Tashkin D P, Kroening R J, Bresler D E, Simmons M, Coulson A H, Kerschnar H 1985 A controlled trial of real and simulated acupuncture in the mangement of chronic asthma. Journal of Allergy and Clinical Immunology 76(6): 855–864
21. Jobst K, McPherson K, Brown V et al 1986 Controlled trial of acupuncture for disabling breathlessness. Lancet Dec 20–27
22. Needham J, Lu G D 1980 Celestial lancets: a history and rationale of acupuncture and moxibustion. Cambridge University Press, Cambridge
23. National Health and Medical Research Council 1974 Report of the working party on acupuncture. Australian Government Publishing Service, Canberra
24. Shanghai Acupuncture Anaesthesia Co-ordinating Group 1972 Why surgical operations are possible under acupuncture anaesthesia. American Journal of Chinese Medicine 1(1): 159–166
25. Peking Children's Hospital 1975 A clinical analysis of 1,474 operations under acupuncture anesthesia among children. Chinese Medical Journal 1(5): 369–374. Also delivered at the 14th International Congress of Pediatrics in Buenos Aires, Argentina, October, 1974
26. Anonymous 1957 Zhonghua Waike Zazhi 5(9): 749
27. Tang D 1984 Principles of the action of acupuncture and moxibustion. Acupuncture Research 3(9): 250–258
28. Chiang C Y, Chang C T, Chu H, Yang L 1973 Peripheral afferent pathway for acupuncture analgesia. Scientia Sinica 16(2): 210–217
29. Brown P E 1972 The use of acupuncture in major surgery. Lancet i: 1328
30. Dimond E G 1971 Acupuncture anaesthesia; Western medicine and Chinese traditional medicine. Journal of the American Medical Association 218(10): 1558–1563
31. Anderson S A, Ericson T, Holmgren E, Lindqvist G 1973 Electroacupuncture effect on pain threshold measured with electrical stimulation of the teeth. Brain Research 63: 393–396
32. Mu J 1985 Paper and lecture presented on the occasion of the Fourth International Advanced Acupuncture Studies program, Nanjing
33. Pomeranz B, Cheng R 1979 Suppression of noxious responses in single neurons of cat spinal cord by electroacupuncture and its reversal by the opiate antagonist naloxone. Experimental Neurology 64(2): 327–341
34. Andersson S A, Holmgren E 1975 On acupuncture analgesia and the mechanism of pain. American Journal of Chinese Medicine 3(4): 311–334
35. Wyke B 1979 Neurological mechanisms in the experience of pain. Acupuncture and Electrotherapeutics Research 4: 27–35
36. Van Nghi N 1972 Acupuncture anaesthesia concerning the first 50 cases conducted in France. American Journal of Chinese Medicine 1(1): 135–142
37. Hillier S M, Jewell J A 1983 Health care and traditional medicine in China 1800–1982. Routledge and Kegan Paul, London.
38. Cheng S B, Ding L K 1973 Practical application of acupuncture analgesia. Nature 242: 559
39. Bannerman R H 1979 Acupuncture: the WHO View. World Health, December, p27–28
40. Fung K P, Chow O K W, So S Y 1986 Attenuation of exercise induced asthma by acupuncture. Lancet Dec 20–27: 1419–1421
41. Berger D, Nolte D 1977 Acupuncture in bronchial asthma: body plethismographic measurements of acute bronchospasmolytic effects. Comparative Medicine: East & West 5(3/4): 265–269
42. Tashkin D P, Bresler D E, Kroening R J, Kerschner H, Katz R L, Coulson A 1977 Comparison of real and simulated acupuncture and isoproterenol in methacholine-induced asthma. Annals of Allergy 39(6): 379–387
43. Takishima T, Suetsugu M, Gèn T, Ishihara T, Watanabe K 1982 The bronchodilating effect of acupuncture in patients with acute asthma. Annals of Allergy 48(1): 44–49

44. Yu D Y, Lee S P 1976 Effect of acupuncture on bronchial asthma. Clinical Science and Molecular Medicine 51(5): 503–509
45. Sliwinski J, Matusiewicz R 1984 The effect of acupuncture on the clinical state of patients suffering from chronic spastic bronchitis and undergoing long-term treatment with corticosteroids. Acupuncture and Electrotherapeutic Research 9(4): 203–215
46. Hyodo M, Gega O 1977 The use of acupuncture analgesia for normal delivery. American Journal of Chinese Medicine 5(1): 63–69
47. Ledergerber C P 1976 Electroacupuncture in obstetrics. Acupuncture and Electrotherapeutics Research 2: 105–118
48. Wallis L, Shnider S M, Palahniuk R J, Spivey H T 1974 An evaluation of acupuncture analgesia in obstetrics. Anesthesiology 41(6): 596–601
49. Tsuei J J, Lai Y, Sharma S D 1977 The influence of acupuncture stimulation during pregnancy: the induction and inhibition of labour. Obstetrics & Gynaecology 50(4): 479–488
50. Zhu R L, Gao X H, Zhou Y L, Yu J 1986 The induction of labour by electroacupuncture stimulation — analysis of 771 cases. In: Zhang X T (ed) 1986 Research on acupuncture, moxibustion and acupuncture anaesthesia. Science Press, Beijing
51. Yip S K, Pang J C K, Sung M L 1976 Induction of labour by acupuncture electrostimulation. American Journal of Chinese Medicine 4(3): 257–265
52. Kubista E, Kucera H, Muller-Tyl E 1975 Initiating contractions of the gravid uterus through electroacupuncture. American Journal of Chinese Medicine 3(4): 343–346
53. Tsuei J J, Lai Y F 1974 Induction of labour by acupuncture and electrical stimulation, Obstetrics & Gynaecology 43(3): 337–342
54. Zhang H Y, Yu L H 1984 Observations on the effect of auriculo-acupuncture for dilatation of cervical os in 56 cases. Second National Symposium of Acupuncture, Moxibustion and Acupuncture Anaesthesia, Paper No 87, Beijing
55. Li H F 1981 The effect of puncturing the Hegu and Sanyinjiao points in pregnancy. Yunnan Journal of Traditional Chinese Medicine 6: 33
56. Sodipo J O A, Falaiye J M 1979 Acupuncture and gastric acid studies. American Journal of Chinese Medicine 7(4): 356–361
57. Matsumoto T, Hayes M F 1973 Acupuncture, electric phenomenon of the skin, and postvagotomy gastrointestinal atony. American Journal of Surgery 125: 176–180
58. Cheng Y Q, Wang Z Q, Zhang S Y, Wu J J, Wu Y W 1984 The use of needling Zusanli in fibroptic gastroscopy. Journal of Traditional Chinese Medicine 4(2): 91–92
59. Omura Y 1975 Pathophysiology of acupuncture treatment; effects of acupuncture on cardiovascular and nervous systems. Acupuncture and Electrotherapeutics Research 1: 511–140
60. Chen K, Liang S, Feng X 1984 The effect of acupuncture using reinforcing and reducing methods on nail microcirculation and local skin temperature. Journal of Traditional Chinese Medicine 4(4): 279–281
61. Li C J, Bi L G, Zhu B J et al 1986 Effects of acupuncture on left ventricular function, microcirculation, cAMP and cGMP of acute myocardial infartion patients. Journal of Traditional Chinese Medicine 6(3): 157–161
62. Lee D C, Lee M O, Clifford D H 1976 Modification of cardiovascular function in dogs by acupuncture: a review. American Journal of Chinese Medicine 4(4): 333–346
63. Lee D C, Lee M O, Jung J W, Tenney T H, Clifford D H 1981 Comparison of the effects of acupuncture at Renzhong (Du 26) and dimethyl sulfoxide (DMSO) on the cardiovascular system of dogs. American Journal of Acupuncture 9(3): 235–242
64. Lee D C, Lee M O, Clifford D H 1974 Cardiovascular effects of acupuncture in anaesthetised dogs. American Journal of Chinese Medicine 2(3): 271–282
65. Lee D C, Lee M O, Clifford D H, Morris L E 1982 The autonomic effects of acupuncture and analgesic drugs on the cardiovascular system. American Journal of Acupuncture 10(1): 5–30
66. Tam K C, Yiu H H 1975 The effect of acupuncture on essential hypertension. American Journal of Chinese Medicine 3(4): 369–375
67. Monaenkov A M, Lebedeva O D, Fisenko L A 1984 Reversal of left ventricular hypertrophy during acupuncture therapy in patients with initial stages of essential hypertension. American Journal of Acupuncture 12(4): 313–320
68. Chui D T J, Cheng K K 1974 A study of the mechanism of the hypotensive effect of acupuncture in the rat. American Journal of Chinese Medicine 2(4): 413–419

69. Lee M O, Lee D C, Kim S, Clifford D H 1975 Cardiovascular effects of acupuncture at St 36 in dogs. Journal of Surgical Research 18(1): 51–63
70. Li P, Sun F Y, Zhang A Z 1983 The effect of acupuncture on blood pressure: the interrelation of sympathetic activity and endogenous opioid peptides. Acupuncture and Electrotherapeutics Research 8: 45–56
71. Han J S, Terenius L 1982 Neurochemical basis of acupuncture analgesia. Annual Review of Pharmacology and Toxicology 22: 193–220
72. Hexum T D, Hanbauer I, Govoni S, Yagb H Y T, Costa E 1980 Secretion of enkephalin-like peptides from canine adrenal gland following splanchnic nerve stimulation. Neuropeptides 1: 137–142
73. Knoll J 1976 Neuronal peptide (enkephalin) receptors in the EAL artery of the rabbit. European Journal of Pharmacology 39: 403–407
74. Bergland R 1985 The fabric of mind. Penguin, Melbourne
75. Cao Q S 1981 Effect of acupuncture on acute myocardial ischemic injury in rabbits. Journal of Traditional Chinese Medicine 1(2): 83–86
76. Chen L B, Li S X 1983 The effects of electrical acupuncture of Neiguan on the PO_2 of the border zone between ischemic and non-ischemic myocardium in dogs. Journal of Traditional Chinese Medicine 3(2): 83–88
77. Liu J L 1984 Role of hypothalamus in the recovery of acute ischemic myocardial injury promoted by electroacupuncture in rabbits. Journal of Traditional Chinese Medicine 4(3): 197–204
78. Meng J 1986 Effect of electroacupuncture on the oxygen metabolism of myocardium during myocardial ischemic injury. Journal of Traditional Chinese Medicine 6(3): 201–206
79. Zhang R, Zhao H 1984 Effect of AQSD resulted from needling in cardiovascular disease. Journal of Traditional Chinese Medicine 4(4): 269–272
80. Zhang H L 1983 Effect of electroacupuncture on the changes in the ECG of acute myocardial ischemic injury in rabbits. Journal of Traditional Chinese Medicine 3(4): 259–264
81. Wu Y X 1982 Therapeutic effect and mechanism of acupuncture at Neiguan (Per 6) in chronic rheumatic heart disease. Journal of Traditional Chinese Medicine 2(1): 51–56
82. Chen S X 1983 Preliminary investigation on the effect of acupuncture of Neiguan (Per 6) and Shaofu (Ht 8) on cardiac function of idiopathic cardiomyopathy. Journal of Traditional Chinese Medicine 3(2): 113–120
83. Mu J, Zhao J Y, Xie S L 1982 Effect of acupuncture on allergic shock of experimental mice. Shanghai Journal of Acupuncture and Moxibustion 3: 195–197
84. Mu J 1985 Influence of adrenergic antagonist and naloxone on the anti-allergic shock effect of electroacupuncture in mice. Acupuncture and Electrotherapeutics Research 10: 163–167
85. He X P, Cao X D, Jiang Y M, Shen L L 1986 Effect of electroacupuncture on electroconvulsive shock in rat: physiological observation and spectral analysis of EEG. Journal of Traditional Chinese Medicine 6(4): 283–287
86. Ionescu-Tirgoviste C, Mincu C 1974 Testing the pancreatic reserve by acupuncture. American Journal of Acupuncture 2(2): 95–101
87. Szczudlik A, Lypka A 1984 Acupuncture-induced changes in human plasma insulin levels. Acupuncture and Electrotherapeutics Research 9(1): 1–9
88. Liao Y Y, Seto K, Saito H, Kawakami M 1980 Effects of acupuncture on the citrate and glucose metabolism in the liver under various types of stress. American Journal of Chinese Medicine 8(4): 354–366
89. Shiryo K 1985 An observation of the effect of acupuncture stimulation on total quantity of 17-OHCS and 17-KS in urine. Proceedings of the Fourth International Congress of Oriental Medicine, Kyoto
90. Wen H L, Ho W K K, Wong H K, Mehal Z D, Ng Y H, Ma L 1978 Reduction of adrenocorticotropic hormone and cortisol in drug addicts treated by acupuncture and electrical stimulation. Comparative Medicine: East & West 6(1): 61–66
91. Wen H L, Ho W K K, Wong H K, Mehal Z D, Ng Y H, Ma L 1978 Changes in adrenocorticotropic hormone and cortisol levels in drug addicts treated by a new rapid detoxification procedure using acupuncture and naloxone. Comparative Medicine: East & West 6(3): 241–245
92. Liao Y Y 1979 Effect of acupuncture on adrenocortical hormone production: (1)

Variation in the ability for adrenocortical hormone production in relation to the duration of acupuncture stimulation. American Journal of Chinese Medicine 7(4): 362–371

93. Brown M L, Ulett G A, Stern J A 1974 The effects of acupuncture on white cell counts. American Journal of Chinese Medicine 2(4): 383–398

94. Hau D M, Guo S T 1985 Comparative study on effects of handling acupuncture, EA and laser acupuncture on counts of various leukocytes in gamma-irradiated mice. Proceedings of the Fourth International Congress of Oriental Medicine, Kyoto

95. Hau D M 1984 Effects of electroacupuncture on leukocytes and plasma protein in the X-irradiated rats. American Journal of Chinese Medicine 12(1–4): 106–114

96. Tykochinskaia E C 1960 Acupuncture as a method of reflex therapy, Voprosy Psikiatriki Nevropatologii, USSR, Vol 7: 249–260, 1960. Secondary source from Hu J H 1974 American Journal of Acupuncture 2(1): 8–13

97. Chu L 1955 Contemporary acupuncture and moxibustion therapy. Xiaohua Publ., Hong Kong. In: Hu J H 1974 Therapeutic effects of acupuncture; a review. American Journal of Acupuncture 2(1): 8–13

98. Qiu M L 1985 Lecture presented on the occasion of the Fourth International Advanced Studies Program in Acupuncture, Nanjing

99. Bresler D E, Kroening R J 1976 Three essential factors in effective acupuncture therapy. American Journal of Chinese Medicine, 4(1): 81–86

100. Sung S K 1976 Mediators of acupuncture. American Journal of Acupuncture 4(1): 25–32

101. Min S Y 1983 Effect of electric acupuncture and moxibustion on phagocytic activity of the reticulo-endothelial system of mice. American Journal of Acupuncture 11(3): 237–242

102. Chu Y M, Affronti L F 1975 Preliminary observations on the effect of acupuncture on immune responses in sensitised rabbits and guinea pigs. American Journal of Chinese Medicine 3(2): 151–163

103. Ding V, Roath S, Lewith G T 1983 Effect of acupuncture on lymphocyte behaviour. American Journal of Acupuncture 11(1): 51–54

104. Gong B, Mo Q Z, Kuang X W, Qian X P, Mao M A, Wang J M, Wang B X 1986 Biochemical and immunological studies on treatment of asthmatic children by means of propagated sensation along channels elicited by meditation. Journal of Traditional Chinese Medicine 6(4): 257–278

105. Selection of the Research Work of Nanjing College of TCM, 1976 College publication.

106. Mu J 1986 The study of acupuncture effect on experimental allergic shock in mice. Acupuncture Research 4: 268–273

107. Bratu J, Stoicescu C 1958 The effects of acupuncture on adrenal glands. Deutsche Zeitschrift für Akupunktur 7: 26

108. Lau B H S, Wong D S, Slater J M 1975 Effect of acupuncture on allergic rhinitis: Clinical and laboratory evaluations. American Journal of Chinese Medicine 3(3): 263–270

109. Schaub M, Fazal Haq M 1977 Electro-acupuncture treatment in psychiatry. American Journal of Chinese Medicine 5(1): 85–90

110. Shi Z, Tan M 1986 An analysis of the therapeutic effect of acupuncture treatment in 500 cases of schizophrenia. Journal of Traditional Chinese Medicine 6(2): 99–104

111. Fischer M V, Behr A, v. Reumont J 1984 Acupuncture — a therapeutic concept in the treatment of painful conditions and functional disorders. Report on 971 cases. Acupuncture and Electrotherapeutics Research 9: 11–29

112. Ceccherelli F, Manani G, Ambrosio F et al 1981 Influence of acupuncture on the postoperative complications following ketamine anaesthesia. The importance of manual stimulation of point R and Shenmen. Acupuncture and Electrotherapeutics Research 6: 255–264

113. Costa C, Ceccherelli F, Ambrsoio F et al 1982 The influence of acupuncture on blood serum levels of tryptophan in healthy volunteers subjected to ketamine anaesthesia. Acupuncture and Electrotherapeutics Research 7: 123–132

114. Shi M S, Zhang J, Cong Y B, Liu R Q, Li B Q, Jia Z P 1986 Experimental study of screening of stimulation parameters of electric needling in acupuncture anaesthesia. In: Zhang X T (ed) Research on acupuncture, moxibustion and acupuncture anaesthesia Science Press, Beijing p 1157–1162

115. Cao X D, Xu S F, Lu W X 1983 Inhibition of sympathetic nervous system by acupuncture. Acupuncture and Electrotherapeutics Research 8: 25–35

116. Zhang A Z, Zeng D Y, Zhang L M, Cheng J S, Ye Z J, Ou S P 1986 Effects of naloxone

on analgesia produced by different strengths of electroacupuncture. In: Zhang X T (ed) 1986 Research on acupuncture, moxibustion and acupuncture anaesthesia. Science Press, Beijing. p 296–302

117. Zhang A Z 1980 Endorphin and acupuncture anaesthesia research in the People's Republic of China (1975–1979). Acupuncture and Electrotherapeutics Research 5: 131–146

118. Nappi G, Facchinetti F, Legnante G et al 1982 Different releasing effects of traditional manual acupuncture and electroacupuncture on propriocortin related peptides. Acupuncture and Electrotherapeutic Research 7: 93–103

119. Sjolund B H, Eriksson M 1979 The influence of naloxone on analgesia produced by peripheral conditioning stimulation. Brain Research 173: 295–301

120. Eriksson M B E, Sjolund B H, Nielzen S 1979 Long term results of peripheral conditioning stimulation as an analgesic measure in chronic pain. Pain 6: 335–341

121. Pomeranz B H, Chiu D 1976 Naloxone blockade of acupuncture analgesia: endorphin implicated. Life Sciences 19: 1757–1762

122. Peets J M, Pomeranz B 1985 Acupuncture-like transcutaneous electrical nerve stimulation analgesia is influenced by spinal cord endorphins but not serotonin: an intrathecal pharmacological study. In: Advances in pain research and therapy No 9: 519–525. Raven Press, New York

123. Cheng R S S, Pomeranz B (1) 1981 Monoaminergic mechanism of electroacupuncture analgesia. Brain Research 215: 77–92

124. Pomeranz B 1986 Relation of stress-induced analgesia to acupuncture analgesia. Annals of the New York Academy of Science 467: 444–447

125. Cheng R S S, Pomeranz B 1979 Electroacupuncture anaesthesia could be mediated by at least two pain-relieving mechanisms, endorphin and non-endorphin systems. Life Sciences 25: 1957–1962

126. He L 1987 Involvement of endogenous opioid peptides in acupuncture anaesthesia. Pain 31(1): 99–121

127. Patterson M A 1975 Addictions can be cured: the treatment of drug addiction by neuro-electric stimulation. Lion Publishing, Berkhamsted

128. Patterson M 1986 Hooked? NET: the new approach to drug cure. Faber and Faber, London

129. Chen Z Q, Xu W, Yan Y S, Chen K Y 1987 Different effects of reinforcing and reducing manipulations in acupuncture assessed by tail flick latency, vocalisation threshold and skin temperature in the rat. Journal of Traditional Chinese Medicine 7(1): 41–45

130. Li C Y, Zhu L X, Ji C F 1987 Relative specificity of points in acupuncture anaesthesia. Journal of Traditional Chinese Medicine 7(1): 29–34

131. Takeshige C 1983 The central mechanism of analgesia in acupuncture anaesthesia — differentiation of acupuncture point and non-point by the central analgesia producing system. Acupuncture and Electrotherapeutics Research 8(3/4): 323–324

132. Lu H C (trans) 1978 The Yellow Emperor's classic of internal medicine and the difficult classic. Academy of Oriental Heritage, Vancouver. The Ling Shu forms part of this text.

133. Rosenblatt S L 1982 Electroencephalogram correlates of acupuncture. American Journal of Acupuncture 10(1): 47–52

134. Varassi G, Manna V, Moffa G, Cassabgi F 1986 Bioelectric brain relations of pain and acupuncture effects on EEG spectral analysis in healthy volunteers. Acupuncture and Electrotherapeutics Research 11: 199–205

135. Shen K F, Ho S F, Wang P F 1986 Effect of cord dorsum stimulation on EEG and behaviour in unrestrained rabbits. In: Zhang X T (ed) 1986 Research on acupuncture, moxibustion and acupuncture anaesthesia.Science Press, Beijing

136. Cahn A M, Carayon P, Hill C, Flamant R 1978 Acupuncture in gastroscopy. Lancet 1: 182–183

137. Wu J L, Zong A M, Chai X M et al 1986 Effects of electroacupuncture on cell-mediated immunity in human body. In: Zhang X T (Ed) 1986 Research on acupuncture, moxibustion and acupuncture anaesthesia. Science Press, Beijing

138. Chang X P 1983 Studies on the mechanism of acupuncture and moxibustion. An-Hui Publishing House, Beijing. (Excerpted by Mu J)

139. National Cooperative Group of Preoperation Forecast of Effectiveness of AA 1986 Comprehensive preoperation forecast of effectiveness of AA and screening of variables. In: Zhang X T (ed) 1986 Research on acupuncture, moxibustion and acupuncture anaesthesia. Science Press, Beijing p 1145–1156

140. Eriksson M B E, Sjolund B H, Nielzen S 1979 Long term results of peripheral conditioning stimulation as an analgesic measure of chronic pain. Pain 6: 335–347
141. Bardychev M S, Guseva L I, Zubova N D 1988 Acupuncture in edema of the extremities following radiation or combination therapy of cancer of the breast and uterus. Vopr Onkol 34(3): 319–322
142. Gerhard I, Postneek F 1988 Possibilities of therapy by ear acupuncture in female sterility. Geburtshilfe Frauenheilkd 48(3): 165–171

FURTHER READING

Hu J H 1974 Therapeutic effects of acupuncture; a review. American Journal of Acupuncture 2(1): 8–13
Hyodo M 1976 The indication of acupuncture in the pain clinic. Presented at the V I World Congress of Anaesthesiology, Mexico City. In: Hyodo M 1977 Recent advances in acupuncture treatment (Part II). Osaka Medical College, Osaka
Kitade T, Toyota S, Morikawa K, Ueki M, Okasaki K, Hyodo M 1976 The study of acupuncture treatment for dysuria in post-radical hysterectomy. In: Hyodo M 1977 Recent advances in acupuncture treatment (Part II). Osaka Medical College, Osaka

3. The nature of the meridians

Because of their intimate involvement in health or the progress of disease, no component of acupuncture theory could be more vital than the meridians (channels) themselves, and they have been a significant area of speculation and research. Enquiry has focused not only on the material basis of meridians (for example, nerve and blood vessel distribution) but also on their less material electromagnetic characteristics. Acupuncture points and their connecting channels may be definable electrically.

The enquiry into the meridians also delves deeply into traditional acupuncture practices. Chinese doctors have argued for centuries that certain parameters of needling are strongly affiliated with the healing outcome. In particular, the propagation of 'Qi sensation', that is, the awareness of warmth, cold, numbness, aching, or tingling radiating from the point of needling along the meridian, is one parameter to which our attention should be drawn. It states in the *Ling Shu*, 'The importance of De Qi lies in the ability to feel the arrival of Qi. The judgement of therapeutic effect depends on it.' And further in the *Zhen Jiu Da Cheng* (Compendium of Acupuncture and Moxibustion) it states, 'In the process of acupuncture, first watch for the approaching of Qi . . . to the point of De Qi. If however, nothing arrives at the end of treatment, healing of disease is not to be expected.'[1]

Does the occurrence of Qi sensation shed any further light on the nature of meridians? Our investigations should not ignore parameters that appear crucial to the practice of acupuncture. We should also look at different needling techniques and note their influence on meridian sensation and their connection with therapy.

It is in these broad areas that this chapter will focus.

ANATOMICAL RELATIONSHIPS OF THE MERIDIANS AND POINTS

In the *Nei Jing Su Wen* it is written that there are 365 acupuncture points, corresponding precisely with the number of days in the year:

Following the course of each of the arteries there are (365) vital points for acupuncture.[2] (p 118)

These channels are deeply imbedded in the muscles; at 365 points, however, they emerge to the surface and thus present the points for needling. The number 365 is significant, for it parallels the days of the year as well as the muscular junctions of the body.[2] (p 62)

This classic number has expanded to as many as one thousand needling sites, especially with the recent development of acupuncture anaesthesia, ear and scalp acupuncture, and other microsystems (foot, nose and hand acupuncture are three common microsystems), all with large numbers of points outside the traditional tracts.[34] The new points that exist now may lead to the rapid disuse of others. Probably fewer than 100 points are commonly used by practitioners today.

Each point has its own traditional name, however, with the rapid growth of new points in the last two decades, naming has not been feasible and a numbering system for the extra points has emerged. Names were chosen historically according to anatomical location or function. For example, Jianwaishu (SI 14) translates as 'Shoulder's outer hollow', whilst Qihai (Ren 6) translates as 'Sea of Qi' reflecting its special function as a source point for Qi.

Besides their names, points were traditionally classified according to physiological function. For example, the five Shu, Antique or Transport points, as they are differently known, have generalised functions particularly on the yin channels. The Jingwell points are used to treat diseases of the viscera and discomfort in the region of the diaphragm and chest. Many other examples could be cited, including the Back-Shu points, Alarm points, and Xi-Cleft points.[3]

Just as the points have been classified according to function, so have the meridians (channels and collaterals). In TCM the meridians are viewed specifically as channels of circulation of Qi and blood. The pulse may be read at various sites along the channels. The channels connect with the internal organs, mutually nourishing and supporting these organs and the superficial tissues. There exist different categories of channels, such as the main tracts with internal pathways (that connect with the internal organs), the transverse Luo mai (that connect the main channels), the longitudinal and fine Luo mai, and the Extra channels. The physiological function of each class of meridian reflects its anatomical distribution. For example, the practitioner wishing to treat an organ disorder would most likely call into action the main tracts with their internal connections, whilst if trying to treat more superficial regions, the longitudinal Luo or Musculotendino channels might be more appropriate. Hence, with clinical use in mind, the Chinese have arrived at a careful systematisation of points and channels. It is totally insufficient to conceptualise the channels simply as lines connecting acupuncture points.

There is a plethora of research relating the channels with anatomical structures. This does not stem solely from a biomedical approach to the understanding of acupuncture channels. The classics themselves make specific references to the anatomical correspondences of the channels[3]:

The twelve primary channels circulate deep within the muscles and cannot be seen. The one that is commonly seen is the Leg Greater Yin (Spleen) Channel as it passes above the inner ankle, since there is no place for it to hide. Those vessels that are commonly seen are all connecting (luo) channels. (*Nei Jing-Ling Shu* Chapter 10) The circulation (within the channels) can be measured externally by palpation of the pulse. After death (the channels) can be seen by dissection. (*Nei Jing-Ling Shu* Chapter 12)[3] (p 111)

Interesting as they are, these attributes referred to in the classics provide little insight in our quest for further understanding of the meridians. For example, it will become apparent later in this chapter that the channels cannot be simply dismissed as a primitive perception of the blood vessels. However, not only has there been investigation of the possible actual anatomical structure of the channels and collaterals, but, as we shall see, some investigators have also focused their attention on the more indirect relationships between the channel and point network and internal anatomy (viscera).

Possible anatomical structure of channels

The dissection of acupuncture points in order to explore the parallels between meridians and the peripheral nerves, blood vessels or lymph vessels would surely be amongst the simplest and most basic of experiments. Yet this rather obvious step, carried out at Shanghai[5] and Harbin,[3] (p 111) would inevitably have to have been performed at some time.

In a series of experiments, acupuncture points were examined for their direct correspondence with nerves, blood and lymph vessels. The Chinese found that out of 324 points examined, 304 were supplied by a superficial cutaneous nerve, 155 with a deep cutaneous nerve, and 137 points were supplied with both. Only 1 point appeared not to be innervated. (Zhang Keren et al provide a thorough morphological study on the receptors of the acupuncture points themselves.)[6]

Amongst 309 points investigated in a different experiment, 24 were shown to lie directly over arterial branches, whilst 262 were within half a centimetre of arterial or venous branches.

In a third experiment only a few points were found to be linked by the same lymph vessel. Most points had no such connection. However, some researchers have noted the significance of lymphatics based on lymphographies and radio-isotope pictures.[7,8] Tiberiu, Gheorghe and Popescu used carbon ink as a radioactive tracer to assess parallels between the lymphatic vessels and the channels.[9] Because of the minimal detail provided by the authors, the significance of the results of these dissection experiments is difficult to assess. It falls into even greater doubt in the light of the more recent French study in 1983 by Simon and colleagues. Simon observed that when the radioactive tracer technetium 99 was injected at an acupuncture point and a control point, transportation away from the points occurred through the lymphatic and venous systems and did not highlight the acupuncture meridians at all.[131]

As regards the meridians on the limbs, there is close correlation between some channels and pathways of peripheral nerves. For example, the lung channel courses its way in a similar fashion to the musculocutaneous nerve, whilst the pericardium channel lies over the median nerve, and the heart channel, the ulnar and medial cutaneous nerve. It should be emphasised, however, that nerves and arteries usually correspond to a very limited part of the channel course.

It is worthwhile considering the relationship between the more modern concept of dermatomes (the somatic segmental character of nerve distribution) and the distribution of the channels and collaterals of acupuncture (Figs 3.1 and 3.2). In many cases channels are contained within the one dermatome for

anterior view   posterior view

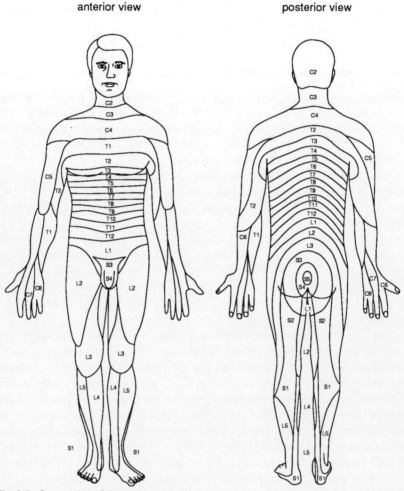

Fig. 3.1 Innervation of dermatone regions.

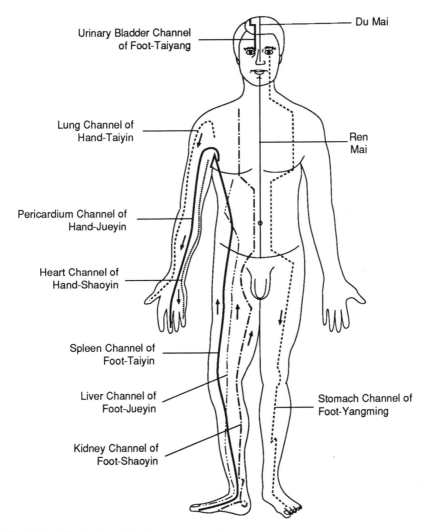

Fig. 3.2A   Distribution of the fourteen channels—anterior view

a considerable part of their length, particularly on the arms and legs. However, despite this overlay, not one meridian could claim to have its pathway restricted to a single dermatome, and certainly, when we contemplate the numerous channels that traverse the trunk, each channel makes contact with multiple dermatomes. Hence, it is apparent that one cannot draw consistent parallels between dermatomal regions and the domains of influence of the acupuncture channels.

Despite this, other evidence illustrates that the functional characteristics of points depends upon the neural segment (dermatome) that they are in. For

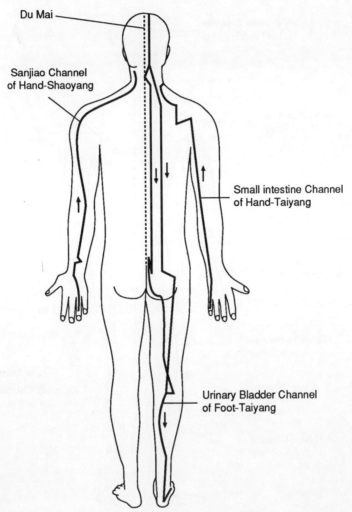

Du Mai

Sanjiao Channel
of Hand-Shaoyang

Small intestine Channel
of Hand-Taiyang

Urinary Bladder Channel
of Foot-Taiyang

Fig. 3.2B   Distribution of the fourteen channels—posterior view

example, the Back Shu points on the Urinary Bladder channel are traditionally named after specific viscera in order to reflect their function and area of influence. Each of these points lies within the dermatome innervating the viscera after which it is named. Curiously, in clinical practice it is also more difficult to obtain 'Qi sensation' (the concept of 'Qi sensation' is discussed in greater detail below) along the Urinary Bladder channel and no apparent reasons for this come forth in the classical literature. This is confirmed by personal experience, and communication with many practitioners and lecturers, including those at the Nanjing College of TCM. Note though, that obtaining sensation along the Ren channel presents far fewer difficulties. Could it be that the dermatome structure, specifically nerve distribution, is significant in the

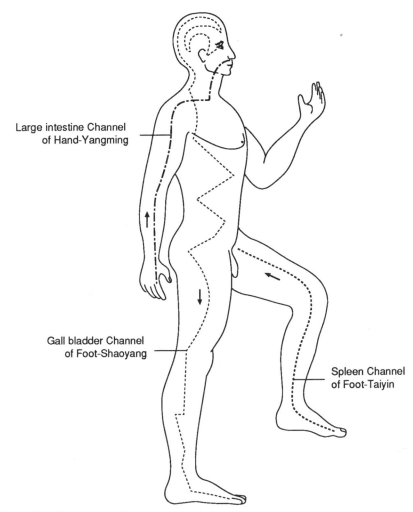

Large intestine Channel of Hand-Yangming

Gall bladder Channel of Foot-Shaoyang

Spleen Channel of Foot-Taiyin

Fig. 3.2C Distribution of the fourteen channels—side view

spread of 'Qi sensation'? Transmission of sensations away from the point of needling would indicate otherwise, as we shall see in many cases described further on.

However, other channels and points corroborate this partial association with the dermatomes. The Hua To Jia Ji points are all located only half to one tsun (a tsun being the standard proportional unit of measurement used to locate acupuncture points) lateral to the median line of the spine, and at the lower end of the spinous process of each vertebra. These points are usually considered to have a function restricted to their dermatomal region of influence. The Extra channel, Dai Mai, or Girdle channel, conspicuously encircles the body and is restricted to between the last thoracic and first lumber dermatome. (There are eight Extra channels which have different passages and functions to the twelve principal channels.) Ren Mai, another Extra channel, illustrates further the case where individual point functions reflect the dermatome in which they are located. A point such as Shanzhong (Ren 17) lies in the fourth thoracic dermatome region and is commonly used for respiratory disorders. Similarly, Zhongwan (Ren 12), in the eighth thoracic is used in gastric conditions, and Guanyuan (Ren 4) in the twelfth thoracic for urogenital disorders. Hence, just as for the Urinary Bladder channel of the back, points on the abdomen and chest may have their functions determined by the dermatome in which they reside.

Nevertheless, such evidence of similarity between meridians and dermatomes does not unite the two under the one title. The two share in part, a common distribution and therefore mutually exhibit certain characteristics. However, there are many cases where a point possesses functions totally separate from what would be expected from its dermatomal distribution. For example, Ganshu (Bl 18), residing in the thoracic region, is used for eye diseases, whilst Fengmen (Bl 12), between the upper portion of the shoulder blades, is adopted frequently in the treatment of a congested nose.[3] Also there are many channels whose pathways, areas of influence, and direction of propagation of 'Qi sensation' are all distinctly separate from dermatomal distribution. Consider channels such as the Small Intestine, Gall Bladder, Stomach, Spleen, and Kidney. Each individually traverses many dermatomes. And 'Qi sensation' may travel in a consistent manner to a region several dermatomes away from the point of needling.

Furthermore, the functions of any group of points are not seen to be even approximately equivalent simply because they reside in the same dermatome, although this may have been implied in the above paragraphs. For example, Shaofu (Heart 8) and Houxi (Small Intestine 3) both lie within the same dermatome but have very varying functions as indicated in the *Essentials of Chinese Acupuncture*:[10]

Shaofu for 'Palpitation, pain in the chest, twitching and contracture of the little finger, feverish sensation in the palm, pruritus, dysuria, enuresis'. (p 159) Houxi for 'Headache, neck rigidity, congestion of the eye, deafness, contracture and twitching of the elbow, arms and fingers, febrile diseases, epilepsy, malaria, night sweating'. (p. 164)

Hence, keeping in mind the significant number of exceptions to the rule, the conclusion must be that there is little evidence to support the claim that channels and points represent physical entities in a common anatomical sense. Although we shall see in subsequent chapters that denervation suppresses the acupuncture effect, we will also witness how simplistic, it would be to assume that the nerves and acupuncture pathways refer to the one and the same thing.

Channels and points as a reflection of internal anatomy

Doubtless the ancient sages were well cognizant of the complex interrelationships between the body surface and internal organs. By palpating along the channels for areas of tenderness a patient's disease could be 'diagnosed'. Identification of these trigger spots, called 'channel diagnosis', gives us some indication of organs involved, but is very crude in that different diseases may cause the same point to react. It is also impossible to identify the stages of a disease. The Front Mu (or Alarm) points are a common classification of acupuncture points that may behave as trigger areas. (Examples of classes of points and specific points that often react as a reflection of internal disorder are provided in most popular acupuncture texts.)[10] However, many such sensitive spots exist outside regular channel points, and therefore have neither category nor name, but are commonly referred to as Ah Shi (Ah yes) points. The existence of these trigger points was acknowledged in the earliest classical texts and formed a considerable part of acupuncture theory in diagnosis and treatment[11] (p 209):

When they are pressed, there should be pain and a sunken sensation. When one wants to determine an acupoint exactly, one should press hard with a finger at one spot after another, then if it is the right one, the patient will feel a relief of his pain (Ling Shu, Ch. 51).

The concepts of trigger points and referred pain are well known to modern medicine and have unfortunately often been promoted as the be all and end all of acupuncture. Referred pain and trigger points probably result from the skin and the viscera sharing the same neural pathways. Perception of referred pain is such that it appears to have originated in the skin rather than the deep seated organ. Felix Mann, in *Scientific Aspects of Acupuncture*, briefly explores these phenomena and concludes that acupuncture treatment operates either through dermatomal (spinal segmental) reflexes or long Sherrington (intersegmental) reflexes.[12] As we shall see, this is hardly the end of the story.

However, in order to be more specific, we should refer to some very interesting experiments relating ear points to internal anatomy. Studies reported by Professor Mu Jian in Nanjing[13] aimed at finding manifestations of duodenal and gastric ulcers in the ears of human and animal patients. By sliding an electrode over the ear surface, numerous sensitive spots were located, which varied in size and shape. (Electroconductivity of acupuncture points is discussed in more detail later in this chapter.)

In 95 cases sensitive spots were tested before, during and after subtotal gastrectomy operations in order to identify patterns of distribution. Sensitive spots on the ear differed according to measurements taken before, during and after the operation. With the progress of the operation and increase of traction force on the internal organs, the number of sensitive spots on the ear rapidly increases, especially in the cavum conchae and on the ear lobe. Clinical observation has shown that the size of the gastric and duodenal ulcer, and the severity of the chronic inflammatory infiltration of mucosa and submucosa, are the main factors determining the number of low resistance spots on the ear. Furthermore, sensitive spots were not confined to a fixed area, nor did they reflect in their distribution in the ear an inverted image of the embryo, a pattern often suggested in ear acupuncture texts. Along with the recovery of the ulcer area, sensitive spots decreased gradually in number.

Similar work was carried out in Beijing Medical College and reported in the Chinese Medical Journal in 1976. The researchers showed that in rabbits, experimentally induced peritonitis and peptic ulcer each led to a significant increase in low electrical resistance points (LERP) in both ears. There was greater correlation of LERP with vascular distribution in the ear, than with vagus nerve distribution.[14]

Under normal physiological conditions, sensitive spots on the auricle should increase in number as long as stimulation of internal organs is continuous. In one study, 346 pregnant women in different stages of pregancy underwent auricular examination.[13] The average number of low resistance spots on the ear altered throughout the term of pregnancy, with the greatest number manifesting immediately prior to labour. During the 2nd and 3rd months of pregancy there were 42 +/−11.7 sensitive spots (50 cases), in the 6th month 20 +/−3.1 (50 cases), in the 7th month 87 +/−18.5 sensitive spots (50 cases), and in the 9th month 125 +/−16.7 (26 cases). Prior to labour there were 167 +/−21.8 sensitive spots (50 cases), whilst 40 days after there were 75 +/−16.2 spots registered amongst 20 cases measured. 6 months after there were 11 +/−4.3 spots on average (20 cases). The principal justification for the alteration of sensitive spots on the auricle during pregnancy is the fact they reflect the increase in volume, weight and tension on the uterus. Endocrine changes are also likely to be implicated, and this issue will be attended to in more detail in Chapter 5.

A completely different approach was devised by Guan Zunxin and reported in the *Yunnan Journal of TCM*.[15] By using a chemical staining solution on the ears of patients suffering from silicosis, Guan Zunxin noticed a significantly higher staining rate of lung points in sick patients than in the control group. Guan Zunxin claims a 95% correlation between this staining method and patients' histories of dust contact with X-ray diagnosis, leading to the claim that this would be a successful form of auricular diagnosis.

RADIATION PHENOMENA ALONG THE CHANNELS

Many believe that the ancients first discovered the therapeutic effects of the acupuncture points and subsequently linked them by lines.[16] However, examination of a meridian silk book that was recently unearthed from a Han tomb at Mawuangdui suggests the reverse. Ancient practitioners may have defined the channels first by observing the phenomenon of propagated sensation.[17]

Needling produces a whole range of sensations which tend to radiate along the channels, away from the point of insertion of the needle. The most common sensations are numbness, distension, aching or soreness, and heaviness. Each occurs more typically in certain regions of the body, as a response to specific needle techniques, and each possesses a variable propensity to radiate.

Numbness is one of the sensations that radiates most readily, followed by soreness and then distension. Soreness appears commonly on the limbs (although not at the extremities, where sharp pain often overides any of the classic sensations) whilst distension is more likely to occur on the trunk. The needling technique of 'setting the mountain on fire', which results in a warming sensation, tends to bring about soreness and distension. The technique of 'cooling like a clear night sky' results in a cooling sensation and numbness. In theory, any sensation may be altered into another with appropriate finger pressing and needle manipulation techniques. Correct breathing, including the art of Qi Gong, can also alter the speed with which Qi sensation arrives at the site of the needle.[18] Finally, the more experience the practitioner possesses, the greater the ease with which these sensations are obtained.

It must be emphasised again how fundamental it is to acupuncture therapy that these sensations are felt by the patient. Quoting the Chinese medical classic, the *Ling Shu* 'When the Qi arrives, the treatment is effective. This is the essential of needling (Ch. 1).' Also, from the *Prose on the Secret of Needling*:

The earlier the arrival of Qi, the faster is the achievement of therapeutic result. Late arrival may signify the failure of treatment. The arrival of Qi is like the sinking and floating of bait caught by a fish. The absence of De Qi is similar to a person spending his boring hours in a vast quiet mansion.[1]

Should such a response fail to arrive then the practitioner is encouraged to reconsider the various parameters of needling such as depth, location and angle of insertion, usage of the pressing hand, and the particular manipulation technique adopted.[19,20,21] The importance of suggestive factors in obtaining Qi sensation were explored by a handful of researchers, all arriving at the conclusion that, no matter how strong a suggestion was given to the patient, it would induce insignificant changes.[22,23]

However, it is not just the patient that is conscious of the arrival of Qi sensation. The physician also often registers a sensation of tightness or drawing on the needle, like a muscular sucking sensation which opposes slightly the withdrawal of the needle. As a consequence of this muscular reaction, physiologists in Shanghai have focused their attention on alterations of electromyogram (EMG) readings.[24,25] These studies performed in China successfully correlated EMG readings with subjective reporting of Qi sensation in both healthy subjects and patients with neuromuscular disorders such as myasthenia gravis, sequelae of infantile paralysis, injury of the brachial plexus, transectional lesions of the spinal cord, amyotrophic lateral schlerosis, myodystrophy, syringomyelia, and taber dorsalis. In all cases of neuromuscular disorders, neither the Qi sensation nor the EMG reading could be aroused.

The only cases where this correlation failed was for myodystrophy, where the electrical responses of the muscles could not be elicited, though the acupuncture sensations seemed to be normal.

Interestingly, in the 15 cases of syringomyelia, a close correlation existed between the degree of loss of Qi sensation and the degree of impairment of pain and temperature sensations, implying that the pathway for the conduction of Qi sensation in the spinal cord is closely related to those for pain and temperature sensations.[13] The direction of transmission of these Qi sensations coincides basically with the direction of circulation and distribution of the channels as recorded in the classics, in contrast to the direction of distribution of nerves. For example, sensation from Guanyuan (Ren 4) should travel down along the Ren channel to the genitals and perineum, traversing as many as three dermatomes.

Research groups from Fujian, Anhui, Shanxi, and Liaoning have completed atlases of channels based on mapping of propagated sensation lines, which were more reliable on limbs than head, (no correspondence), and torso (slight correspondence).[26,27,28] Similar work on the pathways of channel sensation has also been carried out at the Heilongjiang Institute and Guanxi College of TCM.[29] Propagated channel sensations (PCS) have also been found to occur outside China resulting in the calculation of similar maps.[30]

Demonstrations have indicated increased therapeutic results are obtainable if the Qi sensation occurs rapidly on the one hand, and that it reaches the site of disease on the other. (Failing that best results are obtained if the sensation travels as far as possible toward the site of disease.) Up until 1979 most of this work had been limited to analgesia, indicating that an increase in strength and direction of sensation would lead to better analgesic results.[31] Subsequent research has resulted in the extrapolation of these principles to the broad clinical spectrum of acupuncture.[29,32,33] (Many items of related research were presented at the Second National Symposium on Acupuncture and Moxibustion and Acupuncture Anaesthesia (1984), particularly paper numbers 285, 289, 293, and 295.)[34]

In 1984 Shaanxi College of TCM analysed 112 cases of cardiovascular disease. By needling Neiguan (Per 6) and sending sensation up to the chest, their findings suggested that 'acquiring Qi sensation at the site of the disease does not affect improvement of pathological changes and metabolic disturbances of the myocardium...but is mainly successful in alleviating clinical symptoms.'[35] That is, Qi sensation reaching the site of disease is useful in relieving the immediate clinical symptoms (for example, pain and wheezing etc.) but presents to date with insignificant long-term benefits. Note that this is not denying the long-term curative effects of the whole process of acupuncture, but rather the relationship of the cure with the arrival of Qi sensation at the site of the disease. Similar work observing rheographic changes and also using Neiguan (Per 6) has been performed in Shanghai, Beijing, and Baoding, and has been reported in the *Jilin Journal of TCM*.[29,36]

Some investigations show that during acupuncture at Zusanli (St 36), when the propagated channel sensation (PCS) reaches the abdominal area (subjectively indicated by the patient) gastrographs exhibit a decreased frequency and an increase in amplitude in gastric motions. This would be rather unexpected if we were to consider acupuncture working solely through a central neurological action. X-ray observations of peristalsis also highlighted significant differences between persons who were PCS sensitive and to those who were not.[29]

The speed of transmission of acupuncture sensation is far slower than that of nerve conduction. The rate of nerve conduction usually lies between 0.5 and 120 metres per second, depending largely on the class of nerve fibre. Acupuncture sensation, on the other hand, travels with a speed of the order of 10 centimetres per second, which is between 5 and 1200 times slower than the rate of nerve conduction.[37]

Other experiments were initiated in an attempt to observe more objectively the propagated channel sensations in relation to the meridians. Anhui College of TCM tested ten subjects who were all sensitive to propagated channel sensations. Seven out of ten subjects recorded myoelectric potentials along the pericardium meridian, and the amplitudes there were higher than control points either side.[38] Similar experiments were carried out in Hunan[39] and Shanghai[40], confirming strong correlation between recorded muscular activity (EMG's) and local needle sensation (PCS).[41]

The Beijing Institute of TCM recorded temperature changes on the surface of the body via infrared photography.[42] In their experiment they registered distinct dark or bright bands which were correlated to the presence of the propagated channel sensation. EMGs and infrared photography are just two examples of objective measurements of propagated channel sensation. Clinically, skin rashes are also frequently found to be distribute along the pathway of channels.[43,44]

Other experimenters, in their search for objective indices of the meridians, have claimed that sound waves travel more favourably along the meridians, than outside of them.[45] However, contrary to reports in daily newspapers, the results of such experiments still remain debatable.[46,47]

As a consequence of·the investigations into propagated channel sensation, a debate has unfolded for some time over whether this sensation is predominantly a 'peripheral' or 'central' phenomenon. Electromyograms, as mentioned earlier, are one significant piece of evidence that indicates the peripheral nature of this phenomenon. Further evidence to support the fact that PCS is a peripheral excitation also lies in the fact that:

1. The PCS does not follow somatosensory distribution of the nerves in particular regions, for example, the abdomen, and that over a length of the pathway the PCS does not necessarily restrict itself to even one or two dermatomes;

2. Shandong College of TCM (Jinan) showed (in 30 patients with coronary heart disease) that chilling, that is, lowering the temperature of the limb, could block PCS;[48] and

3. Finally, that PCS may be blocked by mechanical pressure.[49,29,41]

Neither chilling nor mechanical pressure is likely to exhibit obvious interference in somatic sensations in the cerebral cortex, but they certainly produce a block in PCS and acupuncture effects. This supports the notion that propagated channel sensation is likely to be a peripheral effect.

In contrast, other investigations argue that the PCS is an excitation that occurs within the central nervous system, although it may be observed peripherally such as in the case of electromyographic responses. In support of this belief is the existence of phantom limb sensation, where the Qi sensation propagates along the meridian on the amputated limb.[50,51] Further observations have been promoted as evidence in support of the central excitation theory, such as on the effect of the local injection of saline, the local or spinal injection of procaine, and spinal sections, all of which prevent (at least our awareness of) the propagated channel sensations.[3,52,53,54] Under lumbar anaesthesia, the subjective Qi sensation felt by the patient, the needle grip response registered by the practitioner, and the EMG changes all disappear entirely in the regions below the level of the anaesthesia.[24] It could be concluded that they involved spinal cord reflexes or mediation to higher centres by way of the spinal cord. In further support, recall the Shanghai researchers already mentioned, who demonstrated that patients with disturbed pain and temperature pathways could not obtain the propagated channel sensation.[25]

The model for 'central excitation' conceives that the impulses from particular points are transmitted to a spinal segment from which they may then travel upward to the brainstem and cerebral cortex, where they are able to generate an awareness of the Qi sensation. Jean Bossy in France proposes that each point communicates with others at the spinal segment level via interneuronal networks of the laminae II and III of Rexed.[8] Somatotopic patterns of communication at this level result in other nerve fibres, not directly stimulated by the needle, transmitting sensation, possibly both centrally to the cerebral cortex and peripherally to the needled region. In addition, the fine fibres of Lissauer's tract, which communicate between adjacent spinal segments, have been suggested as having some responsibility for the development of PCS.[55] Hence, under the model for central excitation, somatotopic organisation at higher levels in the central nervous system may account for the propagated channel sensations (see Fig. 3.3).

ELECTROMAGNETIC PROPERTIES OF THE MERIDIANS

Not only are we able to trace the pathways of propagated channel sensation (via electromyogram and temperature recordings), but the channels themselves may also be identified with measurements of electrical impedance and

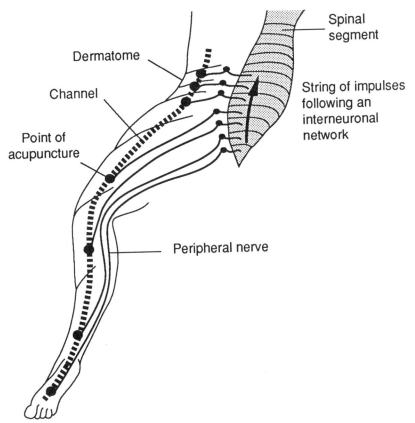

Fig. 3.3 Bossy proposes that somatotopic organisation of somesthetic areas in the central nervous system account for the existence of channels.
(Reprinted with permission from Acupuncture and Electrotherapeutic Research 9(2), 1984; Bossy J, Morphological data concerning the acupuncture points and channel network, 1984.)

conductance.[3,56,57,58,59] In fact, the objective existence of the meridian system is argued most strongly by the electrical specificity of acupuncture points.[60,61] One of the fundamental premises in what I shall hereafter refer to as the 'bioelectric theory of action' is that acupuncture points and channels possess an electromagnetic (EM) characteristic.

The determination of the existence of acupuncture points via electrical means started as early as the 1950s and 60s, particularly with the work of Niboyet in France and Nakatani in Japan.[11,60] By applying a direct current (DC) of 12 volts to the body surface, Nakatani discovered points on the skin of higher conductance than surrounding areas. He subsequently connected these lines with (imaginary) lines of good conductance ('Ryodoraku'), which showed correspondence with the meridians. In later years, the medical colleges of Fujian, Lanzhou and Anhui (China) performed independent research to confirm these results in animals as well as humans.[49,60]

The usual procedure is the application of small external currents to the skin surface, in order to record skin conductance and impedance at specific points in any region. In the cases mentioned above simple direct current (DC) resistance detectors were used, and this was later sophisticated by employing bridge circuitry.[62] Subsequently, alternating current (AC) detectors were introduced in order to prevent polarisation of tissues at the electrode site.

Comparison of various kinds of AC and DC acupuncture point detectors, led some researchers to the claim that high frequency current (200 kHz) is particularly sensitive in identifying acupuncture points.[63] This was confirmed by Fraden and Gelman, who, in studying the physiological effects of electrical parameters on the skin, established that an accurate determination of the electrical resistance could be ensured only when parameters of rather high frequency (above 100 Hz) and very weak electrical current (1 microamp) were adopted.[64]

Using AC bridge circuitry, the electrical resistance between two acupuncture points was determined by Chen and Xie.[65] Interestingly they observed a pattern of variation of resistance corresponding with the 'flux' of Qi described by the 5 Shu (Antique) points. For example, Shangyang (Co 1) has highest resistance and Quchi (Co 11) the lowest. In their experiment they claimed high reproducibility and a low error rate of 4%, despite the pressure of the electrode (5–500 grams) and the time duration spent on the point determining its electrical resistance.

Amongst the dozens of publications in this area, most more rigorous research confirms that there is a significant difference between the electrical identity of true points and nonpoints, with the conclusion that acupuncture points represent *at least an area of high conductivity (electrical permeability) relative to nearby tissues.*[62,66,67,68,69,70,71] For example, Reichmannis, Marino, and Becker assess the AC impedance of part of the meridian with anatomically similar nonmeridian regions and conclude that meridians are electrically distinguishable.[72] However, there are experiments such as those of McCarrol and Rowley, who used a multielectrode grid to show that low skin impedance was only a result of lingering over the same point (and this should be contrasted to the work of Chen and Xie already mentioned).[73]

Some confusion arises from the fact that researchers occasionally determine the impedance between acupoints and the rest of the body, that is, they determine the relative conductivity of a specific point to the whole body. Nordengraaf and Silage attempt to measure the absolute minima in resistance of a point relative to the whole body, rather than determining whether it is a site of low impedance relative to surrounding tissue.[74] Their conclusion was that the value of impedance was so closely related to pressure placed on the electrode, that there is no evidence to support the points as electrically identifiable regions on the surface of the body. In contrast, our first approach, measuring points relative to nearby tissues (devoid of points),[62] suffices to provide an electrical identity of the acupuncture sites, and in fact is likely to be even more accurate, since enormous electrical variability is bound to exist throughout the whole body.

Curiously though, commercial point locators, of which there are many brands on the market (some examples are the Royal Anderson neurometer; Point finder, Model 61–2; Hibiki 7 Japanese Point Finder; Acu Mag Model SX)[75] follow the principles of the second category of study. Specifically they aim to identify the weak impedance of a point relative to the whole body. To devise such sensitive point locators was the goal of most of the early work in France, Japan and China. In a clinical context now, point locators are not infrequently employed, which may be a reflection of their clinical usefulness and success despite the vagaries and inconsistencies raised by Nordengraaf and others.

Studies on the electrical correlates of the meridians and acupuncture points may not only provide insights to the nature and location of the channels and points, but may also claim to be directed at diagnosing illness. Although this is still at a primitive level, some experimenters maintain the degree of electrical impedance on certain channels reflects extant disease processes.[14,82,83,84,85,86,87] Heinrich Voll was one of the earlier Westerners to explore this concept, although he appeared to restrict most of his work to the context of using the Jingwell points.[88,89] In a similar vein other experiments have identified somatic electrical reflections subsequent to surgical operation.[14,79]

Although there is a uniform relationship between sweating and electrical resistance in the skin, this is not sufficient to account fully for the somatic conductance maxima and minima. Many factors have been shown to influence the accuracy of impedance measurements including the emotional state of the patient, the degree of sympathetic discharge, the skin moisture factor, the thickness and local pathology of the skin, and the possibility of vagotonia.[90] The Shanghai acupuncture text claims that skin electricity reflects autonomic nervous function and is related to the opening and closing of the pores,[3] but others disagree and see more complex relationships involved.[70,91]

Unfortunately, even if we acknowledge the relationship between illness, sweating and skin electricity, this still sheds no light on the reason for the patterns of distribution of sensitive spots on the ear during illness or after surgery as discussed earlier in this chapter. It is clear that the electrical resistance of acupuncture points on the surface of the body will vary in response to numerous factors such as pathological changes in the viscera;[76] or other illnesses;[77] as a consequence of sleep or physical activity; as a response to changes in the external environment, for example, the weather and time of day;[78] or after nerve intervention or needling of points.[79,80,81] It is interesting to note also that the amount of electroconductivity shows a broad relationship with anatomical location, specifically the head, then trunk, then the limbs manifest higher electroconductivity, and that this does not necessarily correlate with areas of injury or profuse sweating.[3]

Other evidence, which tentatively corroborates our electromagnetic (EM) theory of the existence of the channels and points, is the application of Kirlian photography. Kirlian photography basically involves the use of a high voltage, low amperage, radio frequency, alternating current acting between two capacitance plates. When the small current is discharged onto a specimen and the photographic film placed between the two electrode plates, it is believed the resultant photographic image represents a bioplasmic pattern particular to the specimen, that is the presence of an ion 'aura' around the specimen. In the context of acupuncture, some researchers have claimed they can recognize illness, measure the benefit of treatment, and identify the presence of points and channels, all via Kirlian photography.[92,93,94,95,96,97] Others, however, appear justified in their claim that the evidence is still rather flimsy.[98,99]

Many other experiments have attempted to assess the significance of bio-electric emanations from acupuncture points and channels (such as the use of radioactive tracers),[9] but because they are generally single experiments, they do not currently present a strong argument.[101,102]

THE BIOELECTRIC THEORY OF ACTION

Except possibly for the work of Reichmannis, Marino and Becker, there has been nothing that constitutes a substantial theory of acupuncture based upon the bioelectric properties of the channels and the bioelectric responses to treatment.[62,66,72,103] However existing information can be integrated to form a de facto theory of action. The three premises that follow below imply that needling is able to influence physiological function, and therefore health and disease, electromagnetically. This, I will argue, may be considered the primary mode of action of acupuncture, whilst the neurological responses discussed in Chapters 4 and 5 have a secondary position, that is, they occur as a result of changes in electromagnetic field patterns and strength in the region of needling.

The basic premises of this 'bioelectric theory of action' would be roughly as follows:

1. **Points and channels exhibit an electromagnetic nature.** This has already been fully discussed in the pages above and acknowledges the electrical identity of acupunture points and channels and their measurement with various devices in both health and disease.

2. **Needling induces alterations in the electromagnetic properties of the channels and tissues.** Some evidence is provided that electromyographic activity is present during acupuncture and correlates highly with the acupuncture sensation[24,25,100,105] This sensation is known to travel extensively away from the site of needling. Hence, needling may produce electrical changes along the channels, and it has been stated earlier that the action of needling alters the electrical resistance of the points. Approaching the problem in a different way, Ionescu-Tirgoviste and Popa illustrated that tonification and dispersal techniques can be distinguished by ionic changes in the vicinity of the needle.[106] And finally this leads us to our third premise.

3. Electromagnetic fields significantly influence biological matter and physiological functions.

The influence of electromagnetic fields on biological matter and physiological functions is well documented. The adoption of small electric fields to enhance wound healing dates back as far as the 17th century with the application of gold leaf to lesions, resulting in an electrostatic influence which is believed to be responsible for the tissue healing.[107]

In 1792 Galvani observed that injured tissues generated small electric currents. When the electrical balance of the body is disturbed in an injury, the resulting shift in current flow (referred to as the 'current of injury') triggers a biological repair system. As healing continues, the direct current potential difference approaches the normal electrical balance relative to the surrounding tissues. These electrical phenomena have been measured by Lund in plants,[108] by Becker in bone,[109] and by Wolcott and associates in soft tissue.[107,110]

Robert Becker has been one of the pioneering investigators in this area of bioelectric potentials. Becker proposes the existence of a complete direct current (DC) electrical system which controls basic functions such as growth, regeneration, biological cycles and tissue repair.[104] This DC system also 'interlocks with the nervous system and is postulated to be its precursor'. Becker summarises some of his work as follows:[104]

It is known that DC potentials measurable on the intact surfaces of all living animals demonstrate a complex field pattern that is spatially related to the anatomical arrangement of the nervous system. The surface potentials appear to be directly associated with some element of the nervous system and they can be measured directly on peripheral nerves themselves where they demonstrate polarity differences depending upon whether the nerve is primarily motor or sensory in function. (p 188)

Furthermore, Becker goes on to say that these and other observations:

would appear to indicate that the action potential system existed upon a substratum of DC potentials which may have antedated the action potentials as a mechanism of data transmission. If this is so, then the pre-existing DC potentials must have had originally, and may still have, control functions over basic properties of living organisms. Such a function has been determinmed in the case of the reaction to injury and the self repair processes that follow it. (p 189)

External electric currents may also be adopted to encourage repair and growth. This was shown in bone repair,[111] growth in higher plants[112] and by the inhibition of bacterial growth in vitro.[113] Other researchers have examined the effect of electric currents on more specific physiological functions such as adenosine triphosphate (ATP) generation, protein synthesis and membrane transport.[114]

More recently, two researchers have been at the forefront of news for their work on cancer. Bevan Reid of Sydney University focuses on the manner in which electromagnetic fields influence crystal growth and biological change.

Through study specifically on cervical cancer, he has found that cancer cells exhibit a different 'energic' pattern in terms of the way light is diffracted through them.[115,116,117] These electromagnetic patterns are, it would appear, an expression of cell dysplasia, and hence normal or dysplasic cells may also be vulnerable to influence by electromagnetic fields.

On the other side of the world in Sweden, Bjorn Nordenstrom makes similar claims in the context of lung cancer. He has undertaken the treatment of lung cancers by electrotherapy, whereby he inserts one needle into the tumour, and another nearby, and between them applies a small DC electric current in order to change the polarity of charge distribution within the tumour.[118] Other scientists have also observed distinct corona discharges as a result of altered electronic properties and photon emission of tumours.[119]

Furthermore magnetism and laser are often used in therapy, and laser has been more recently adopted in the context of acupuncture. Attempts have been made to measure magnetic fields around humans,[120] and many reports exist on magnetic treatment and subsequent physiological change[68,121,122,123,124] Although laser is used for a variety of conditions,[125] the mechanism by which it works on cell tissue is still rather elusive.[126,127,128] However, laser has been shown to produce changes in cell polarisation, local tissue currents and neural activity.[129,130] Laser affects tissues directly, but also obviously influences the acupuncture meridians by its broad therapeutic applications. It is important to note here that electromagnetic changes in somatic regions may have an influence on the internal viscera by neural connection or otherwise.

The fact that acupuncture meridians and points possess an electrical nature, combined with the observations of the influences of small electric currents on tissues, can only serve to reinforce the proposal that needling, by altering the electrical field in the immediate vicinity, may bring about more widespread physiological changes. The evidence discussed in this chapter on the nature of the meridians lends further credibility to Becker's proposal that DC potentials may interlock with the nervous system, and in fact be its morphological precursor. Data transmission through the DC potential system need not be radically different to the communication along acupuncture meridians.

REFERENCES

1. Cheung C S (trans) 1983 Notes on de qi. Journal of the American College of Traditional Chinese Medicine 1: 66–67. Originally appeared in Pu Y R 1980 Zhong Yi Zha Zi 6
2. Veith I (trans) 1966 Huang Di Nei Jing Su Wen (The Yellow Emperor's classic of internal medicine). University of California Press, Berkeley ch. 1–34
3. Shanghai College of Traditional Chinese Medicine 1981 Acupuncture – a comprehensive text. O'Connor J, Bensky D(trans). Eastland Press, Chicago
4. Lo C K 1981 Nose, hand and foot acupuncture. Commercial Press, Hong Kong
5. Huang D K 1983 Relationship between the points of channels and peripheral nerves. Acupuncture & Electrotherapeutics Research 8(3/4): 328
6. Zhang K 1982 A morphological study on the receptors of acupuncture points. Journal of Traditional Chinese Medicine 2(4): 251–260

7. Gong Q H, Xiang Y M, Cao J R, Wang W J, Wei H X 1985 Studies on the relationship between the channels and the lymphatic system. TCM Digest vol 1(2)
8. Bossy J 1984 Morphological data concerning the acupuncture points and channel network. Acupuncture & Electrotherapeutics Research 9: 79–106
9. Tiberiu R, Gheorghe G, Popescu I 1981 Do meridians of acupuncture exist? A radio-active tracer study of the bladder meridian. American Journal of Acupuncture 9(3): 251–256
10. 1980—The essentials of chinese acupuncture Foreign Languages Press, Beijing
11. Needham J, Lu G D 1980 Celestial lancets—a history and rationale of acupuncture and moxibustion. Cambridge University Press, Cambridge
12. Mann F 1983 Scientific aspects of acupuncture. Heinemann Books, London
13. Mu J 1984 Lecture presented at the Fourth Advanced Acupuncture Studies Program, Nanjing, China.
14. Acupuncture Anaesthesia Research Group, Beijing Medical College 1976 Survey of electrical resistance of rabbit pinna in experimental peritonitis and peptic ulcer. Chinese Medical Journal, New Series, 2(6): 423–434
15. Guan Z X 1981 A new method for the research on ear acupuncture—staining of auricular points. Yunnan Journal of Traditional Chinese Medicine, 5: 27. Abstract also appears in TCM Digest, Vol 1(1): 55
16. Guan H H, He Z M, Wu H T 1979 The formation and development of 'channel theory'. National Symposium of Acupuncture and Moxibustion and Acupuncture Anaesthesia, Beijing Paper No 248
17. Meng Z W 1979 The origin, establishment and prospect of the theory of channels. National Symposium of Acupuncture and Moxibustion and Acupuncture Anaesthesia, Beijing Paper No 247
18. He Q, Zhou J, Yang B, Zhao G, Zhai T, Liu Y 1984 Researches on the propagated sensation along meridians excited by Qigong. Second National Symposium of Acupuncture and Moxibustion and Acupuncture Anaesthesia, Beijing Abstract No 280
19. Research group of acupuncture anaesthesia and channels, Guangxi College of Traditional Chinese Medicine 1986 Propagated sensation along the channels(PSC) induced by stimulation of ear points. In Zhang X T (ed). Research on acupuncture, moxibustion, and acupuncture anaesthesia. Science Press, Beijing
20. Wang B X, Cui L H, Chu W Z 1986 Phenomenon of propagated sensation along the channels induced by limitation of spontaneous activity (entering quiescient condition). In: Zhang X T (ed) Research on acupuncture, moxibustion, and acupuncture anaesthesia. Science Press, Beijing
21. Zhang J, Liu W C, Wang T, Cheng K M, Yu S Z, Zhang R X 1986 Preliminary study of excitation of propagated sensation along channels. In: Zhang X T (ed) Research on acupuncture, moxibustion, and acupuncture anaesthesia. Science Press, Beijing
22. Hu X L, Wu B H, You Z Q, Chen D L, Li B J 1984 Studies on the role of hint in the formation of the propagated sensation along meridians. Second National Symposium on Acupuncture and Moxibustion and Acupuncture Anaesthesia, Beijing Paper No 342
23. Yuan C X, Yan C Y 1984 Observation of propagated sensation along meridians (PSM) phenomena of 250 cases under strong suggestion. Second National Symposium on Acupuncture and Moxibustion and Acupuncture Anaesthesia, Beijing Paper No 343
24. Acupuncture Anaesthesia Group, Shanghai Institute of Physiology 1973 Electromyographic activity produced locally by acupuncture manipulation. Chinese Medical Journal 9: 118 (English summary)
25. Department of Physiology of Shanghai First Medical College and Acupuncture Anaesthesia Co-ordinating Group of Hua Shan Hospital, Shanghai 1973 Acupuncture sensation and EMG of the needled point in patients with nervous diseases. Chinese Medical Journal 10: 137 (English summary)
26. Anhui, Fujian, Shanxi, Liaoning Cooperative Group 1979 Studies on the propagated sensation lines of the 14 channels. National Symposium of Acupuncture and Moxibustion and Acupuncture Anaesthesia, Beijing Paper No 253
27. Meng Z W, Liu W Z, Chen M X, Wang S, Lu C Y 1984 New charts on 14 meridians. Second National Symposium of Acupuncture and Moxibustion and Acupuncture Anaesthesia, Beijing Paper No 264
28. Ji Z 1981 Studies on propagated sensation along the channels. Journal of Traditional Chinese Medicine 1(1): 3–6

29. Meng Z, Zhu Z, Hu X 1984 New development in the researches of meridian phenomena in China during the past five years. Acupuncture Research 9(3): 207–222
30. Zhang R X 1984 Determination of the phenomena of propagated sensations along meridians on the bodies of Guineans. Second National Symposium of Acupuncture and Moxibustion and Acupuncture Anaesthesia, Beijing Paper No 271
31. Cooperative Group in Research of PSC, Fujian Province 1986 Studies of relation between propagated sensation along channels and effectiveness of clinical acupuncture analgesia. In Zhang X T (ed) Research on acupuncture, moxibustion, and acupuncture anaesthesia. Science Press, Beijing
32. Gong B, Mo Q H, Kuang X W et al 1986 Biochemical and immunological studies on treatment of asthmatic children by means of propagated sensation along channels elicited by meditation. Journal of Traditional Chinese Medicine 6(4): 257–278
33. Wu S H, Sheng L L, Gu P K, Yang H Y, Tie S Y 1986 Study of objective parameters in phenomenon of propagated sensation along channels. In: Zhang X T (ed) Research on acupuncture, moxibustion, and acupuncture anaesthesia. Science Press, Beijing
34. Second National Symposium of Acupuncture and Moxibustion and Acupuncture Anaesthesia, 1984, Collection of abstracts. All China Society of Acupuncturists (Publ), Beijing
35. Zhang R, Zhao H 1984 Effect of AQSD resulted from Neiguan needling in cardio-vascular disease; analysis of 112 cases. Journal of Traditional Chinese Medicine 4(4): 269–272
36. Liu G J 1981 The observation on the changes of rheography in 311 cases by activating the channel Qi. Jilin Journal of Traditional Chinese Medicine 3: 12. Abstract also appears in TCM Digest vol 1(1): 56
37. Meng Z W 1984 A new approach to the theory of the meridians—theory of the third equilibrium and theory of holographic informations from regions. Second National Symposium of Acupuncture and Moxibustion and Acupuncture Anaesthesia, Beijing Paper No 263
38. Xing J H, Yuan C X, Zhang F Q 1984 EMG analysis of dominant propagated sensations along meridians in normal subjects. Second National Symposium of Acupuncture and Moxibustion and Acupuncture Anaesthesia, Beijing Paper No 312. Also reported in Acupuncture Research 3(9): 217, 1984.
39. Yan J, Yi S X, Wang L H et al 1984 An observation of muscular electricity of 'propagated sensation along the meridian'. Second National Symposium of Acupuncture and Moxibustion and Acupuncture Anaesthesia, Beijing Paper No 311
40. Guo W Y, Sun T T, Zhou S X, Tang X S, Lu G Z 1984 The computerised analysis of the EMG signals of needling reaction in acupuncture. Second National Symposium of Acupuncture and Moxibustion, and Acupuncture Anaesthesia, Beijing Paper No 313
41. Research Group of Acupuncture Anaesthesia, Fujian 1986 Studies of phenomenon of blocking activities of channels and colllaterals. In: Zhang X T (ed) Research on acupuncture, moxibustion, and acupuncture anaesthesia. Science Press, Beijing
42. He G, Shu Q, Shi J, Zou L, Zhang S 1984 Objective view of the channels via infra-red thermography. Second National Symposium of Acupuncture and Moxibustion and Acupuncture Anaesthesia, Beijing Paper No 318
43. Li D Z 1986 Existence of channel system as evidenced by 93 cases of skin diseases appearing along the channels. In: Zhang X T (Ed), Research on acupuncture, moxibustion, and acupuncture anaesthesia. Science Press, Beijing
44. Wu Y, Liu A, Chen Y 1984 Preliminary observations on the changes of cutaneous temperature on the acupoints along meridians caused by acupuncture. Second National Symposium of Acupuncture and Moxibustion and Acupuncture Anaesthesia. Beijing Paper No 314
45. Sing Tao Jih Pao (Beijing newspaper) 17 April 1987
46. Zhu Z X, Xie J G, Ding Z M et al 1984 Study on the specific percussion sound of the line of latent propagated sensation along meridians. Second National Symposium of Acupuncture and Moxibustion and Acupuncture Anaesthesia, Beijing Paper No 323
47. Chen M X, Xu G S, Wang K M, Ouyang S, Wang H Z, Zhu W F 1984 Experimental studies on the detection of acoustic emission signals for propagated sensation along meridians. Second National Symposium of Acupuncture and Moxibustion and Acupuncture Anaesthesia, Beijing Paper No 328

48. Xiao Y J, Su D G 1984 Effect of local refrigeration on ECG changes of EA in Neiguan acupoint. Second National Symposium of Acupuncture and Moxibustion and Acupuncture Anaesthesia, Beijing Paper No 291
49. Fujian Institute of TCM 1959 Approach to the problem of the nature of meridians Journal of Chinese Medicine (10): 9
50. He G X 1984 Observation and analysis on the phenomenon of propagated sensation along the meridians in 52 amputees. Second National Symposium of Acupuncture and Moxibustion and Acupuncture Anaesthesia, Beijing Paper No 341
51. Li B N, Wang D S, Hu C 1984 A primary analysis of propagated hallucination along meridians in 55 amputees. Second National Symposium of Acupuncture and Moxibustion and Acupuncture Anaesthesia, Beijing Paper No 340
52. Lu C Y 1984 Comparative studies on the correspondence between the dominant and recessive propagated sensations along meridians. Second National Symposium of Acupuncture and Moxibustion and Acupuncture Anaesthesia, Beijing Paper No 270
53. Ernst M, Lee M 1983 Sympathetic effects of manual and electrical acupuncture of Hegu and Zusanli points as evidenced by thermography. Acupuncture & Electrotherapeutics Research 8(3/4) (Abstract only)
54. Fu Z M, Li B N, Xiao Z J 1986 Preliminary observations on propagated sensation along channels in 102 cases of spinal cord transection. In: Zhang X T (ed) Research on acupuncture, moxibustion, and acupuncture anaesthesia. Science Press, Beijing
55. Shenyang Medical College 1973 Preliminary experimental morphologic and electron microscopic studies of the connection between acupuncture points on the limbs and segments of the spinal cord. Chinese Medical Journal 3: 34
56. Zhu Z H, Yan Z Q, Yu S Z et al 1986 Studies of phenomenon of latent propagated sensation along the channels: 1 The discovery of a latent PSC and preliminary study of its skin electrical conductance. In: Zhang X T (ed), Research on acupuncture, moxibustion, and acupuncture anaesthesia. Science Press, Beijing
57. Yu S Z, Zhang R X, Zhou D, Zhu Z X, Xie J G, Xu R M 1984 The measurement of latent PSM lines along the meridian of hand shaoyang and the determination of its cutaneous electric resistance. Second National Symposium of Acupuncture and Moxibustion and Acupuncture Anaesthesia, Beijing Paper No 302
58. Xie J G, Xu R M, Yu S Z, Huang S F, Zhu Z X 1984 Experimental localisation and the low impedance nature of the line of latent propagated sensation along meridian of the stomach. Second National Symposium of Acupuncture and Moxibustion and Acupuncture Anaesthesia, Beijing Paper No 303
59. Liu Y M, Zhu Z X, Yu S Z, Xie J G, Fu X M, Huang S Y 1984 Determination of the low impedance nature of the line of latent propagated sensation along the meridian of large intestine by 3 skin impedance detectors. Second National Symposium of Acupuncture and Moxibustion and Acupuncture Anaesthesia, Beijing Paper No 304
60. Zhu Z X 1981 Research advances in the electrical specificity of meridians and acupuncture points. American Journal of Acupuncture 9(3): 203–216
61. Becker R O, Reichmannis M, Marino A A, Spadaro J A 1976 Electrophysiological correlates of acupuncture points and meridians. Psychoenergetic Systems 1: 105–112
62. Reichmannis M, Marino A A, Becker R O 1975 Electrical correlates of acupuncture points. Institute of Electrical and Electronics Engineers Transactions on Biomedical Engineering, Nov. p 533–535
63. Ghaznavi C 1974 Localisation of acupuncture loci by electrical impedance measurements. Proceedings of the Second New England Biomedical Engineering Conference, Worcester Polytech, 387. Sited from Zhu Z X 1981 (see Biblio No 60 above)
64. Fraden J, Gelman S 1979 Investigation of nonlinear effects in surface electroacupuncture. American Journal of Acupuncture 7(1): 21–30
65. Chen W, Xie J 1979 A new method for the determination of the superficial electrical resistance of the points. National Symposium of Acupuncture and Moxibustion and Acupuncture Anaesthesia, Beijing Paper No 294
66. Reichmannis M, Marino A A, Becker R O 1976 DC skin conductance variation at acupuncture loci. American Journal of Chinese Medicine 4(1): 69–72
67. Bossy J 1984 Sensory potentials evoked by stimulation of the jing points at the hand. Acupuncture and Electrotherapeutics Research 9: 195–201

68. Prince J P 1983 The use of low strength magnets on EAV points. American Journal of Acupuncture 11(2): 125–130. Reports that the polarity of magnets could influence the speed of bone repair, pain intensity, bleeding rate and other physiological functions.
69. Zhu Z X, Huang S F, Xie J G et al 1984 The observation of low impedance line along meridian of rat. Second National Symposium of Acupuncture and Moxibustion and Acupuncture Anaesthesia, Beijing Paper No 306
70. Zhu Z X, Huang S F, Xie J G, Yu S Z, Xu H M 1984 Observation of the low impedance line along meridian of rabbit before and after anaesthesia and bleeding. Second National Symposium of Acupuncture and Moxibustion and Acupuncture Anaesthesia, Beijing Paper No 307
71. Zhang L S, Tang Y Z, Zhang Z X 1984 Study of the skin impedance of the commonly used acupoint in sheep. Second National Symposium of Acupuncture and Moxibustion and Acupuncture Anaesthesia, Beijing Paper No 308
72. Reichmannis M, Marino A A, Becker R O 1979 Laplace plane analysis of impedance on the heart meridian. American Journal of Chinese Medicine 7(2): 188–193. (Showed that impedance between two Heart channel points was significantly lower than between two adjacent non-meridian points. This supports the idea that meridians are likely to be an information transmission system different from the nervous system.)
73. McCarrol G D, Rowley B A 1979 An investigation of the existence of electrically located acupuncture points. Institute of Electrical and Electronics Engineers Transactions on Biomedical Engineering 26(3): 177–181
74. Noordergraaf A, Silage D 1973 Electroacupuncture. Institute of Electrical and Electronics Engineers Transactions on Biomedical Engineering 20: 364–366
75. Cracium T, Berindean I 1978 Acupuncture apparatus for point location, EA and transcutaneous analgesia. American Journal of Acupuncture 6(3): 229–233
76. Wu X J 1979 Observation of the connection between viscera and body surface—the acupuncture point reaction in 105 cases with diseases of the stomach and liver. National Symposium of Acupuncture and Moxibustion and Acupuncture Anaesthesia, Beijing Paper No 293
77. Kuang P G, Hou W K, Shi X C, Li H, Xiao Y S 1979 Preliminary investigations on the relation between headache and electrical conductive capacity of acupuncture points on the auricle. National Symposium on Acupuncture and Moxibustion and Acupuncture Anaesthesia, Beijing Paper No 292
78. Ionescu-Tirgoviste C 1975 Anatomical and functional particulates of the skin areas used in acupuncture. American Journal of Acupuncture 3(3): 199–206
79. Matsumoto T, Hayes M F 1973 Acupuncture, electrical phenomenon of the skin, and postvagotomy gastrointestinal atony. American Journal of Surgery 125: 176–180
80. Research Laboratory of the Mechanisms of Acupuncture Anaesthesia, Morphology Group, Beijing Medical College 1986 Adrenergic nerve fibres—the chief factor affecting changes of electric resistance of rabbit pinna in experimental peptic ulcer. In: Zhang X T (ed) Research on acupuncture, moxibustion, and acupuncture anaesthesia. Science Press, Beijing
81. Yin H Z, Zhou S C, You G F 1986 Experimental study of the afferent pathway in formation of low resistance points on the auriclae of rabbit. In: Zhang X T (ed) Research on acupuncture, moxibustion, and acupuncture anaesthesia. Science Press, Beijing
82. Ionescu-Tirgoviste C, Constantin D, Bratu I 1974 Electrical skin resistance in the diagnosis of neurosis. American Journal of Acupuncture 2: 247–252
83. Bergsmann O, Woolley-Hart A 1973 Differences in electrical skin conductivity between acupuncture points and adjacent skin areas. American Journal of Acupuncture 1(1): 27–32 (They showed that when the electrical potential rose to around 10 volts, the nonlinear turning point of the voltage-current curve known as the threshold current could be established as an index to register the low resistance of acupuncture points.)
84. Tsuei J J 1984 A food allergy study utilising the EAV acupuncture technique. American Journal of Acupuncture 12(2): 105–116
85. Ionescu-Tirgoviste C, Bajenaru O 1984 Electric diagnosis in acupuncture. American Journal of Acupuncture 12(3): 229–238
86. Kobayashi T 1984 Cancer diagnosis by means of Ryodoraku neurometric patterns. American Journal of Acupuncture 12(4): 305–312
87. Ionescu-Tirgoviste C 1985 The electric potentials of jing distal points in diabetes with and without polyneuropathy. American Journal of Acupuncture 13(1): 5–14

88. Voll R 1975 Twenty years of EA diagnosis in Germany. American Journal of Acupuncture 3(1): 7–17
89. Voll R 1987 Verification of acupuncture by means of electroacupuncture according to Voll (EAV). American Journal of Acupuncture 6(1): 5–15
90. Madill P 1984 Uses and limitations of acupuncture point measurements, German EA or EAV. American Journal of Acupuncture 12(1): 33–42
91. Hu J H 1974 Therapeutic effects of acupuncture: a review. American Journal of Acupuncture 2(1): 8–14
92. Kightlinger J F 1974 Organ system pathology diagnosis by kirlian photography of digit acupuncture terminal points. American Journal of Acupuncture 2(4): 258–265
93. Wei L Y 1975 Brain response and Kirlian photography of the cat under acupuncture. American Journal of Acupuncture 3(3): 215–223
94. Poock G K 1974 Statistical analysis of the bioluminescence of acupuncture points. American Journal of Acupuncture 2(4): 253–257
95. Luciani R J 1978 Direct observation and photography of electroconductive points on the human skin. American Journal of Acupuncture 4(6): 311–317
96. Johnson K 1975 Photographing the non-material world. Hawthorn Books, New York.
97. Krippner S, Rubin D (eds) 1974 The Kirlian aura: photographing the galaxies of life. Anchor Books, New York
98. Schaar W W van der 1976 Organ pathology diagnosis and acupuncture. American Journal of Acupuncture 4(3): 252
99. Lin X Z, Li G Q, Lu W X, Guan Y 1984 Observations on kirlian photography oh biliary tract cases taken prior and subsequent to the operations. Second National Symposium of Acupuncture and Moxibustion and Acupuncture Anaesthesia, Beijing Paper No 321
100. Yan J, Yi S X, Wang L H et al 1986 An observation of muscular electricity of 'propagated sensation along the meridian'. Second National Symposium of Acupuncture and Moxibustion and Acupuncture Anaesthesia, Beijing Paper No 311
101. Giller R M 1975 Chi energy and bioelectric phenomena. American Journal of Acupuncture 3(4): 342–346
102. Yan Z Q 1983 A study on the pathological illuminating signal point investigation of 300 subjects. Journal of Traditional Chinese Medicine 3(1): 37–40
103. Becker R O 1974 The basic biological transmission and control system influenced by electrical forces. Annals of the New York Academy of Sciences 238: 236–241
104. Becker R O 1974 The significance of bioelectric potentials. Bioelectrochemistry and Bioenergetics 1: 187–199
105. Guo W Y, Sun T T, Zhou S X, Tang X S, lu G Z 1986 The computerised analysis of the electromyographic signals of needling reaction in acupuncture. Second National Symposium of Acupuncture and Moxibustion and Acupuncture Anaesthesia, Beijing Paper No 313
106. Ionescu-Tirgoviste C, Popa E 1986 Tonification and dispersion effect of an acupuncture needle obliquely introduced into an electric field. American Journal of Acupuncture 14(4): 339–343
107. Carley P J, Wainaple S F 1985 Electrotherapy for acceleration of wound healing: low intensity direct current. Archives of Physical Medicine and Rehabilitation 66: 443–446
108. Lund E J 1925 Experimental control of organic polarity by electrical current: nature of control of organic polarity by electric current. Journal of Experimental Zoology 41: 155–190
109. Becker R O 1967 Electrical control of growth processes. Medical Times 95: 657–669
110. Wolcott L E, Wheeler P C. Hardwicke H M, Rowley B A 1969 Accelerated healing of skin ulcers by electrotherapy: preliminary clinical results. Southern Medical Journal 62: 795–801
111. Bassett C A L 1974 Augmentation of bone repair by inductively coupled electromagnetic fields. Science 184: 575
112. Gensler W 1974 Bioelectric potentials and their relation to growth in higher plants. Annals of the New York Academy of Science 238: 280–299
113. Rowley B A, McKenna J M, Chase G R, Wolcott L E 1974 The influence of electrical current on infecting microorganism in wounds. Annals of the New York Academy of Science 238: 534–551

114. Cheng N 1982 The effects of electric currents of ATP generation, protein synthesis, and membrane transport in rat skin. Clinical Orthopaedics and Related Research 171: 264–272
115. Reid B L 1986 Propagation of properties of chemical reactions over long distance in the atmosphere as seen by crystal growth pattern changes. Australian Journal of Medical Laboratory Science 7 (Feb): 30–35
116. Sydney University News 18(22), 1986
117. Reid B L 1985 The causation of cervical cancer (Parts 1 and 2). Clinics in Obstetrics and Gynaecology 12(1): 1–32
118. Taubes G 1986 An electrifying possibility. Discoverer, April: p22–37
119. Rein G 1985 Corona discharge photography of human breast tumour biopsies. Acupuncture and Electrotherapeutics Research 10: 305–308
120. Payne B 1984 A new device which detects and measures an energy field around the human body. American Journal of Acupuncture 11(4): 353–358
121. Prince J P 1983 Further experience with low strength magnets applied to EAV acupuncture points. American Journal of Acupuncture 11(3): 249–254
122. Schuldt H 1978 Body potential and electroacupuncture in amputation pains and internal organ functions. American Journal of Acupuncture 6(2): 103–106.
123. Hsu M, Fong C 1978 The biomagnetic effect: its application in acupuncture therapy. American Journal of Acupuncture 4(6): 289–296
124. Rose-Neil S 1979 Acupuncture and the life energies. ASI Publishers, New York
125. Kleinkort J A, Foley R A 1984 Laser acupuncture: its use in physical therapy. American Journal of Acupuncture 12(1): 51–56
126. Zalesskiy V N, Belousova 1 A, Frolov G V 1983 Laser acupuncture reduces cigarette smoking. Acupuncture and Electrotherapeutics Research 8: 297–302
127. Trelles M A, Rotinen S 1983 He/Ne laser treatment of haemorrhoids. Acupuncture and Electrotherapeutics Research 8: 289–295
128. Tang H, Fu Y D 1981 Helium-Neon laser irradiation of acupuncture points in treatment of 50 cases of acute appendicitis. Journal of Traditional Chinese Medicine 1(1): 43–44
129. Olson J E, Schimmerling W, Tobias C A 1981 Laser action spectrum of reduced excitability in nerve cells. Brain Research 204: 436–440
130. Uzdensky A B 1982 On selectivity and locality of the effects of laser microirradiation of cells. Cyotology 24(10): 1110–1133
131. Simon J, Guiraud G, Esquerre J P, Lazorthes Y, Guiraud R 1988 Acupuncture meridians demystified. Contribution of radiotracer methodology. Presse Medicale 17(26): 1341–1344

FURTHER READING

Hu X, Wu B, You Z et al 1986 Preliminary analysis of the mechanism underlying the phenomenon of channel blocking. Journal of Traditional Chinese Medicine 6(4): 289–296
Baker D W 1984 An introduction to the theory and practice of German EA and accompanying medications. American Journal of Acupuncture 12(4): 327–332
Brown M L, Ulett G A, Stern J A 1974 Acupuncture loci: techniques for location. American Journal Of Chinese Medicine 2(1): 67–74
Schuldt H 1981 The application of nosodes in EAV. American Journal of Acupuncture 9(2): 161–164

4. Paradigms of the biomedical action of acupuncture

If any distinctive theme pervades research on acupuncture it is the attempt to fit this elusive therapy into western biomedical paradigms. Acupuncture initially met with disbelief amidst cries of 'placebo' and 'hypnosis', but this response has been gradually superseded by the neurological paradigm. However, despite the scale of recent research, suggestions that placebo and hypnosis are the beginning and end of acupuncture still exist.[1]

The neurological paradigm conceives of acupuncture working through mechanical nerve contact, with all influences transmitted via neural pathways. This view initially took form in Melzack and Wall's 'gate control theory' in 1965 (see Ch. 5). It subsequently prompted the attention of sympathetic researchers whose work aimed at confirming the hypothesis that acupuncture only operated within dermatomal regions, and thereby endorsed the principles of the gate control theory as originally presented. In 1973 Chinese investigators found that there existed a significant humoral component during acupuncture therapy.[2] This once again led to a wave of research in the West, with experiments on endocrine and blood changes. An appropriate paradigm shift followed to incorporate the concept that therapy was at least partly a result of humoral influences.

Another theme seems to be an attempt to remain as true as possible to the concept of 'Qi', however interpreted.[3] This line of investigation explores the bioelectric phenomena of the channels and points, and even the possible ways in which the neural or humoral response might occur as a result of initial bioelectric influences. The thesis is still limited to certain scientific circles in Eastern Europe, Asia and some Scandinavian countries.

So many paradigm shifts in such a short span of investigation suggests a fertile approach to research. However, even a cursory look at the changes in direction indicates that these rapid shifts stem more from initial lack of knowledge, and better awareness later, of the nature and characteristics of acupuncture therapy. For example, Melzack's gate control theory was developed initially with only a spinal gate in mind. However, traditional teaching about acupuncture points includes far more than a segmental neural response. To the Chinese empiricist, the early gate control theory was incomplete. This also happened with research that confined acupuncture to dermatomal influences, or limited it to the concept of a double gate theory, and so on.

77

Information regarding the nature and characteristics of acupuncture therapy is not new to this decade, and has existed for hundreds of years, but research questions regularly fail to incorporate this knowledge.

The distinct neurological and humoral models mentioned above, rapidly blended to form a more generalised 'neurohumoral' paradigm, and researchers have emphasised either the humoral or neural aspects of this paradigm to suit their needs. The weight placed on the neurohumoral thesis by researchers is a reminder of the one-dimensional thinking predominant in the West. The acceptance of the neurohumoral theory can be accounted for if we examine history.

President Nixon's trip to China in 1972 brought to the West a glimpse of acupuncture in action—surgery carried out under acupuncture anaesthesia. That highly impressed Nixon's entourage of doctors. In the eyes of the West it represented the pinnacle of success for acupuncture. As surgical anaesthesia was the issue, no great conceptual leaps were required to see that it was the result of neural interference that was being observed. Investigators already had their sights directed—acupuncture must affect nerve pathways. These beginnings still influence most research.

Yet the neurohumoral paradigm falls short in its ability to explain some aspects of acupuncture. It has failed to address the importance of point specificity, a case that has been clearly represented by the work of Takeshige and others.[4,5] There is no reason contained within the neurohumoral hypothesis as to why acupuncture works well at a particular locus or possesses specific therapeutic indications there, yet may induce a negligible change just one centimetre away, although the sham locus still is within the same area of nerve distribution. The sham locus may even be richer in blood vessels and nerve distribution.

Other than a handful of researchers exploring the concepts of neurohumoral mediators, few have tackled the relationship between 'Qi sensation' and the value of treatment. This is no small aspect of acupuncture therapy. Appropriate 'Qi sensation' is closely correlated to the success of acupuncture. This has also been verified experimentally.[6,7] Differences in the skill of the practitioner also warrant attention, especially in the light of the large number of current studies that do not acknowledge the importance of needling experience.

Despite these drawbacks there is considerable sophistication in neurohumoral research into acupuncture (as will shortly become evident) but to suggest that we have arrived at an acceptable 'mechanism of action' is premature. The ultimate measure of the credibility of any scientific model lies in its ability to predict consequences of experimental or natural situations. The neurohumoral model lacks the ability to specify the use of any points for particular diseases. On the other hand the Chinese have had available a theory providing guidance on treatment for thousands of years (for example, 5 Phase (Element) theory defines the functions of the Antique-Shu points). The inability to correlate the needling of specific acupuncture loci with results is the most significant shortfall of the neurohumoral concept.

Current western medical research, it appears, has been more fruitful in accounting for the gamut of effects brought about by acupuncture therapy than predicting the result of its application. Many theories are on offer, and most explain the treatment of specific diseases.[8,9] No one theory is capable of accounting for the broad effects of acupuncture and but few theoretical proposals can be discarded completely.

The success of acupuncture therapy has all too often been dismissed as the result of either placebo, hypnosis, stress analgesia, or ethnic differences. None account for the variety of success acupuncture has and it is worthwhile illustrating some of the relevant research which should have buried these theories.

Acupuncture therapy has an outstanding record of clinical effectiveness. It has succeeded in some cases where all other therapies have failed. This ancient medical procedure does require more thorough explanation, but this should not be a barrier to its adoption in the western health care system. Research, however, needs to be directed more clearly to define the limitations of acupuncture technique and produce guidelines that act more successfully as predictors of its efficacy. There is very little information to date on this.

The placebo effect

A placebo factor does exist in acupuncture just as with all types of medical intervention. However acupuncture offers more than simply a placebo response. This is endorsed by many experiments which have attempted to measure the placebo effect by of stimulating nonpoints.[4,5,10,11,12,13] Many investigators exploring analgesia or other physiological responses have used nonpoint acupuncture on control groups to calculate the effective placebo. Other experiments involved needling real points without giving electrostimulation,[14,15] needling real points that were inappropriate to the treatment,[16] attachment of inert surface electrodes,[17] holding down experimental animals, or even carrying out double blind studies where the practitioner himself did not know the value of the chosen points.[11,14,18] The majority of this research significantly endorses the value of true acupuncture over sham, with the real acupuncture groups responding markedly better.

Takeshige[4,5] in 1983 and 1985 confirmed some earlier work[10] to conclude that stimulation of correct acupuncture points is imperative to cause significant acupuncture analgesia, while nonpoint stimulation causes insignificant analgesia, which is also different in nature. He went on to illustrate that acupuncture analgesia differs from nonacupuncture analgesia, (that is, acupuncture stimulation but not at an actual acupuncture point), in several ways[4]:

Acupuncture analgesia:
1. lasts for a long time after cessation of stimulation (aftereffect),
2. exhibits individual variation in effectiveness, and
3. is completely blocked by naloxone, but not by dexamethasone (a glucocorticoid).

On the other hand…non-acupuncture analgesia:
1. decreases gradually after a definite time during stimulation,
2. has no individual variation in effectiveness, and
3. is blocked by dexamethasone but not by naloxone. (p 323)

As chemical nerve inhibitors are capable of distinguishing between acupuncture and nonacupuncture treatments, there must exist differing pharmacological, and therefore neurological, pathways. Although Takeshige found the descending pain inhibitory system to be the same for real and placebo treatment, the afferent pathways differed. The weight given to the placebo effect is certainly diminished in the light of experiments that indicate the importance of needling real loci. But there is other evidence to undermine the placebo claim (as the only effect of acupuncture).

With repeated use a placebo becomes less effective, in contrast to acupuncture therapy. It is generally observed in China and elsewhere that greater frequency of acupuncture treatment only improves the result. (Some experiments repeat treatment until a certain pattern of response has been obtained and the placebo effect thereby diminished. Data uncontaminated by the placebo effect is then collected).[19] Furthermore a placebo is not likely to work when no relief has been obtained with many other forms of therapy, a stage most western patients have reached by the time they opt for acupuncture. This is especially so if morphine and other analogues have already been tried and proved unsuccessful. Natural opiates have been shown to be involved in placebo analgesic responses, however they are not likely to exhibit much potency during acupuncture if the morphine analogues were ineffective in earlier therapy.

There are other inconsistencies. Experimenters in Shanghai have shown that needling on a limb where circulation has been occluded results in the same pain threshold rise as needling without occlusion of circulation, a fact which does not fit the concept of placebo analgesia.[2] The whole field of veterinary acupuncture also sheds considerable doubt on the validity of the placebo, as animals are not likely to be aware of the positive purpose of needle insertion, although no doubt stress responses warrant consideration here.

Claims have been made that the exotic nature of acupuncture acts strongly in its favour to produce a placebo response, however, as Kaptchuk has already argued, this is hardly likely in the case of the Chinese where results using their home medicine are no less effective than other forms of therapy, and if anything only reflect a greater expertise than in the West due to the quality of experience and training.[20]

Placebo acupuncture can at least in part induce a release of endogenous opiates and hence influence analgesia, drug withdrawal, and other disorders to some degree.[21,22] It would appear sensible to incorporate as baseline in future clinical studies the placebo effect and distinguish it from pure acupuncture results, a suggestion already proposed by Joseph Needham.[23 (p 261)] Individual differences in experimental subjects may prove this too complex an option, in which case acupuncturing nonpoints or inappropriate acupuncture points would represent a satisfactory form of control.

Finally, many other characteristics peculiar to acupuncture need to be borne in mind. In placebo acupuncture it should not matter what point is needled on the surface of the body, all having a relatively equivalent influence. Yet the very fact that acupuncture loci are electrically definable, as mentioned in Chapter 3, emphasises the importance of meridian theory. As such it not be surprising that needling an identifiable point would achieve a more specific result than needling a random point on the skin. Similarly, different frequencies of stimulation or manual manipulation techniques produce different results, a fact not easily reconcilable with a placebo effect. Furthermore, over 20 neurotransmitters have been found to be involved in the acupuncture effect, including many hormone substances.

And so the evidence mounts. Clearly placebo has an influence but is far from the full picture. Clinical studies that still make such claims need to be scrutinised very closely as regards their definitions and techniques, and ultimately, whether true acupuncture was performed.

Hypnosis

Most of the issues raised with the placebo concept could be raised again in the context of hypnosis, although the majority of work here has focussed on comparing hypnotic analgesia to acupuncture analgesia. There is a multitude of observations that really do not lend much support to the hypnosis hypothesis. But one of the most powerful arguments is that whilst acupuncture analgesia is reversible by naloxone, hypnotic analgesia is not, indicating that a different mechanism is operating.[24] Different states of awareness of the patient are also exhibited.

Many mediators, (neurotransmitters in particular), are engaged more fully during acupuncture than hypnosis, and the efficacy of acupuncture shows a close correlation with the release of these mediators. Surgery under hypnotic analgesia is considered viable in 10% to 14% of the population, in contrast to acupuncture anaesthesia, which may be workable in as much as 80% to 90% of the population.[23 (p 239)] The significance of this is that there is 70% of population for whom acupuncture analgesia works, yet hypnotic analgesia does not.

Animals, children and babies can be treated successfully with acupuncture but are not easily hypnotised.[25,26,27] At the Beijing Children's Hospital acupuncture analgesia has been used on children from 4 months to 14 years old with good success. Although some operations were easier than others, the overall effectiveness was claimed to be approximately 80%.[28]

On the other hand, work by Knox and Shum found that patients who are more susceptible to hypnotism are also more likely to be responsive to acupuncture, which suggests at least some common mechanisms.[24] In contrast other researchers have found that the degree of susceptibility in different individuals had nothing to do with the effect of acupuncture analgesia.[29]

Stress analgesia

It has long been established that the application of a variety of noxious and/or stressful manipulations result in the development of analgesia, both opiate and nonopiate.[30,31,32] The whole domain of physiological pain relieving systems is vast. Multiple analgesic systems exist, including the opiates and nonopiates, and each system may be called into action dependent upon the variables of stimulation, such as region,[4] duration, frequency[33,34] and intensity.[35,36]

Obviously the question arises as to how much of acupuncture therapy or, more specifically, analgesia, is a result of stressful intervention? Despite the amount of conflicting information in stress induced analgesia and acupuncture research, some specific and consistent observations may be selected and highlighted in order to illustrate the difference between the two.

Zhang Anzhong (1980)[37] and Bruce Pomeranz (1986)[38] are two of the only investigators who attempt to address this question throughly. In brief, Pomeranz points out that:

1. Sham acupuncture (needles placed in nonacupuncture points) fails to produce analgesia whereas true acupuncture (needles placed in true points designated by Chinese atlases) produces analgesia in awake animals[39] and human subjects.[40] Both sham and true acupuncture produce the same amount of stress. (Similar work was also performed by Takeshige.[5])
2. Electroacupuncture given at three different frequencies in awake rodents produces different effects, yet all three should be equally stressful. At 0.2 Hz no analgesia was observed.[41] At 4 Hz there is an analgesia mediated by endorphins.[39,41] At 200 Hz there is an analgesia mediated by serotonin.[42] Similar results have been observed in humans.[33]
3. Acupuncture in awake horses releases cortisol. However sham acupuncture has no cortisol effect even though it should be equally stressful.[43]
4. Finally, that acupuncture analgesia is targeted to specific painful sites. For example, stimulation of Hegu (Co 4) produces analgesia of the face and neck, but not of the lower extremities.[44] Stress induced analgesia should produce analgesia over the entire body equally in a fight or flight response. (p 444)

Zhang also mentions a plethora of observations that distinguish acupuncture analgesia from stress induced analgesia. For example, in one experiment assessing the effect of naloxone on acupuncture analgesia produced by different strengths of electrostimulation, it was observed in rabbits that under weak intensity stimulation the plasma cortisol and cAMP levels were normal or low, and that the analgesic response could be reversed by naloxone.[45] However, under stronger stimulation the animals struggled, the plasma cortisol and cAMP rose, and the analgesia was not reversed by naloxone. From this experiment it could be concluded that the mechanism of stress analgesia, that is, the stronger stimulation which causes the animals to struggle, differs from moderate strength acupuncture, where the analgesia is partially a result of the activity of opiate receptors.

Zhang, summarising some of the recent Chinese literature makes the following claims[37]:

1. Acupuncture analgesia (AA) is naloxone reversible, but stress analgesia (SA) is not. Some authors have reported that SA could be partially antagonised by large doses of naloxone, twenty times higher than that for reversing AA, thus suggesting that even if there are endorphin factors involved in SA, they might act on different opiate binding sites.
2. During AA, plasma cAMP level decreases and plasma cortisol level remains normal both in human beings and rabbits; but these two biochemical indices markedly increase during SA.
3. The central grey is essential for the AA effect, but not for SA.
4. Using radioimmunoassay, it was found that changes of enkephalins content during AA are quite different from that during SA.
5. Dorsolateral spinal cord lesions eliminated AA but not SA, which could be abolished by spinal transverse dissection, suggesting that the descending pathway essential for AA is different from that for SA. (p 143)

There seems little doubt that acupuncture treatment adds up to much more than a stress response.

Medical anthropologists have explored cultural components related to pain and have gone so far as to measure the response between some ethnic groups. Zborowski[46], and Josey and Miller[47] all found that cultural origin was significant in any individual's tolerence to pain.[23(p236),48] Other fascinating research is reported in textbooks of medical anthropology, where it is illustrated that culture determines the very nature of complaints and symptoms that are expressed by a patient.[49] For example, Jenyi Wang details the somatization of symptoms in Chinese culture as a means of circumventing cultural inhibitions of presenting with emotional or psychological disorders.[50] In the context of pain sensitivity and acupuncture, these findings are further endorsed by studies on genetic variations in animals. Peets and Pomeranz observed that a specific breed of mice, deficient in opiate receptors, were not as responsive to acupuncture analgesia, and concluded that 'presumably some patients might be genetically more susceptible to acupuncture than others.[51] Interestingly enough such genetic variations were also noticible in the context of stress induced analgesia.[52]

Hence it may prove fruitful for medical anthropologists and researchers to explore further the ethnic and cultural complexities of acupuncture.

THE NEUROHUMORAL PARADIGM

Research into what mediates the acupuncture effect has directed our attention into three broad areas:

1. *Neural mediation* which incorporates the concept that nerve fibres carry and transmit the acupuncture and is confirmed largely by experiments which test the acupuncture influence after denervation in the region of

needling, nerve section, or interference with neural transmission of the acupuncture impulse:

2. *Humoral mediation* which includes communication of the acupuncture effect via the circulation of neurotransmitters and other hormones in the blood stream and cerebrospinal fluid; and

3. *Bioelectric mediation* which is a theory that maintains that the meridians are electrically distinct and that changes in them act as precursers to neurological and humoral responses.

In this section I will address the research relating to the first two areas only. A preference for adopting the concept of either neural or humoral mediation depends largely on the physiological context being explored. For example, if investigating the acupuncture treatment of an endocrine disorder, it would be sensible to begin with measurements of blood hormone changes subsequent to treatment. On the other hand, when exploring the analgesic responses to acupuncture, it is a logical step to consider the role of nerve distribution and interaction of neural impulses. However, the predominance of either neurological or humoral influences is difficult to gauge and their perceived relevance to any disease is largely dependent upon the medical models of the time. Richard Bergland explores this cogently in his recent publication *The Fabric of Mind*.[53] He presents a strong case for discarding the antiquated paradigm of the brain as a dry electrical organ operating like a computer. Instead Bergland proposes that the brain behaves more like a gland in the way it releases, and is influenced by, hormones. Hormonal codes may travel to and from the brain, and the brain, therefore, shares influence with all parts of the body. The process of thinking, which in the past has been considered strictly neurological, is a consequence of hormonal action not only in the brain but all over the body.

If we relate Bergland's concept back to the range of influences produced by acupuncture, it is not difficult to conceptualise acupuncture as a technique which orchestrates hormonal symphonies. Despite the significant overlap between the domains of neurological and hormonal influences, the concept of a harmonious 'symphony' may be a helpful tool in understanding how acupuncture works. But first we should turn our attention more to research that defines the neurological mechanisms behind acupuncture.

Neural mediation

Modern neuroanatomical knowledge relates in distinct ways to the acupuncture system. The existence of referred pain, trigger points, and somatovisceral reflexes, all linked into the theory of dermatomes, is significant as evidence of the connection of cutaneous areas of the body with the viscera. It also suggests the possible neural pathways of the acupuncture model, as somatic stimulation, at least at a segmental level, may be able to treat visceral disorders. That the Chinese were aware of these possibilities early in their investigations is substantiated by the many experiments that monitor visceral responses to the acupuncture stimulation of cutaneous areas of the body.[23(p 209)54,55]

However, comparative studies by various researchers on the role of Lissauer's tract and intersegmental reflexes provide evidence that dermatomes are flexible in their boundaries and associated segmental spinal levels[56,113] Furthermore, actual clinical experience of acupuncture therapy indicates that treatment responses, analgesic or otherwise, are not restricted to operating within segmental, or neighbouring segmental, levels, contrary to the conclusion propounded by many researchers including Needham and Lu[23] and MacDonald.[56]

In acupuncture analgesia it has become more and more evident that the needles must be placed in the same dermatome as the surgical intervention. (Needham and Lu, p 207)

The insertion of the acupuncture needles in the region (painful area) or others sharing the same segmental supply is more likely to produce a beneficial effect with less stimulation than inserting them elsewhere. (McDonald, p 278)

The use of Hegu (Co 4) for dental analgesia could be forced into this restricted segmental concept. The use of other points, however, such as Guangming (GB 37) for eye diseases, or Houxi (SI 3) for low back pain, and the ear points Lung and Shenmen as the most successful for chest analgesia[57] are some of the evidence that does not support the segmental spinal concept as the principal neuroanatomical pathway involved in the acupuncture response.

Acupuncture analgesia is effective on the head and the face and areas which are not supplied by any segmental spinal nerve, hence the inhibitory effect of acupuncture must be possible at different levels of the central nervous system, such as the spinal cord, brainstem, and limbic system. This helps explain anomalies regarding point selection that are puzzling in the light of dermatome theory.

There appears little doubt that an intact functioning nervous system is required at all times for acupuncture to induce analgesia, or, for that matter, any physiological changes in the subject. Specifically, section of the principal nerve innervating a region will result in placement of the acupuncture stimulus there having no effect whatsoever.

Studies in Nanjing found that if rabbit limbs were denervated by removal of the femoral and sciatic nerves prior to needling, no analgesic effect would be observed.[58] Similar results were also obtained in Pennyslvannia.[25,59] Nerve sections are also responsible for obstructing the more general physiological effects of acupuncture. For example, Needham reports on some interesting personal observations of experiments in Shanghai.[23] In these studies, which concerned experimental appendicitis in dogs, he states:

The tip of the caecum was tied off and a mixed culture of staphylococci and streptococci injected into it; then acupuncture treatment was given, and the tissues of both treated and control animals removed for histological analysis on the fourth day. Inflammation was very heavy in the latter and light to medium in the former. Partcularly interesting was the fact that if the dorsal sympathetic ganglia and the trunk with its roots was cut on both sides between the 5th and 12th segments the protective function of the acupuncture was completely inhibited. (p 202)

Approaching from a different perspective, it is apparent that interference with circulation does not prevent the analgesic effect of acupuncture. Shanghai physiologists Chiang and colleagues illustrated that vascular occlusion of the upper limb in a group of volunteers did not stop acupuncture induced analgesia.[2] Needling an acupuncture locus on the hand below the level of the vascular occlusion (with a tourniquet) still induced the same analgesic response (as measured by rise in pain threshold) at a distant target site.

After introducing local anaesthetic both deeply and cutaneously, these physiologists also concluded that the deep, as opposed to superficial, nerve receptors were responsible for transmission of the acupuncture stimulus. It appeared that the afferent impulses for acupuncture analgesia are transmitted mainly via the deep nerves. It is also worthwhile noting that the superficial nerve block did not inhibit the Qi sensation either, whilst the deep block did.

Certain experiments performed on cats in Nanjing Medical College involved the bilateral transection of the dorsal and lateral funiculi to observe the role of these nerve tracts in transmission of the analgesic effect of acupuncture.[58] Transection below the spinal level of incoming acupuncture impulses brought no change, whilst transection above did. It was found that the central afferent pathway in acupuncture analgesia follows the lateral funiculus of the spinal cord, particularly the anterolateral part, (otherwise commonly known as the spinothalamic tract, although also includes the spinoreticular tract).[60] Transection of the dorsal funiculus (lemniscal pathway), on the other hand, appeared to have no significant effect on acupuncture analgesia. This was also confirmed by Levy and Matsumoto who claimed that the lemniscal system is not strongly involved, if only because the animal's proprioceptive function seems unaltered with acupuncture analgesia.[25]

We are already beginning to touch on the general concepts of afferent and efferent inhibition of pain signals by acupuncture. Afferent inhibition of pain refers to the modulation of pain information as a consequence of the interaction of ascending impulses from the site of pain with those due to stimulation from the acupuncture point. This afferent interaction may occur at various levels of the central nervous system with the result of diminuation of the pain sensation. Efferent inhibition, on the other hand, refers to acupuncture analgesia brought about as a direct consequence of the influence of descending neural pathways on the ascending (afferent) pain impulses. Both afferent and efferent inhibition have a role to play in the management of pain, and therefore it is likely that they are also involved in other physiological responses to acupuncture.

Afferent impulses arising from the site of pain may interact at various levels of the central nervous system with those impulses derived from the point of acupuncture. That is, inhibitory gates are possible at different levels of the neuroaxis, resulting in the modulation of pain information. Chang Hsiangtung illustrated that this inhibition may occur in the thalamus, specifically in the nucleus parafascularis and the nucleus centralis lateralis[61]:

Experiments performed in albino rats and rabbits showed that certain neurons in nucleus parafascicularis (Pf) and also nucleus centralis lateralis (CL) of thalamus could give rise to characteristic unit discharges in response to nocuous stimuli, and these discharges...were concerned with pain. Pain responses of the Pf and CL neurons could be inhibited by electrical needling of certain acupuncture points, squeezing the Achilles tendon or weak electrical stimulation of a sensory nerve. Too strong stimulation, however, tended to exaggerate the response to pain. (p 25)

Chang's experimentation further suggested that the efficacy of acupuncture for analgesia is determined mainly by the state of brain excitability. Similar work by Shen, Tshai and Lan illustrated that inhibitory gating actions are present in the brainstem.[62] (see Ch. 5).

Acupuncture analgesia is also strengthened by descending or efferent inhibition. The pathway of descending inhibition appears to be located in the dorsolateral (corticospinal) portion of the spinal cord, transection of which may result in elimination or attenuation of the analgesic effect of acupuncture below the transected level.[58] As early as 1973, Anderson had concluded that the gradual onset and decline of the pain threshold implied the existence of a descending control system in electroacupuncture analgesia.[63]

So far we have mainly discussed the mechanical severing of nerve pathways in order to test the subsequent potency of acupuncture. There are other tools which have been used to map the neurological action of needling. Chemical blockers may be introduced, for example, in the form of antagonists to particular neurotransmitters, and consequently obstruct neural pathways. As an example, naloxone, a morphine antagonist which takes up receptor sites to the natural opiate neurotransmitter substances in the body, when introduced subcutaneously or intrathecally, will suppress the analgesic effect caused by needling. This provides important evidence that the naturally occurring opiate like substances in the body, (neuropeptides such as endorphins and enkephalins), act as neurotransmitters in nerve pathways at least in the context of acupuncture analgesia.[4,39,64]

At this stage it is worth clarifying the role of neurotransmitter substances and their receptor sites. Neurotransmitters act to communicate one neurone with another, to carry a signal on in a sequential fashion to its targeted region (see Fig. 4.1). Responding to the catalyst of a nerve signal impulse, neurotransmitters are released from the synaptic vesicles (contained in the pre-synaptic knob of Neurone 1), and travel across the synaptic cleft to take up receptor sites on the post-synaptic membranes, thereby exciting or inhibiting Neurone 2.

Each neurone produces and releases only one single type of neurotransmitter substance. These neurotransmitters will have a positive or negative modulating influence on the nerve impulse depending on the nature of the uptaking receptors. Note that Figure 4.1 illustrates a more complex involvement where Neurone 3 has a presynaptic influence on the normal Neurone 1 to 2 pathway. In this case an impulse travelling along Neurone 3 will cause a release of enkephalins which will in turn inhibit the release of acetylcholine (Ach) and thereby suppress the impulse travelling along from Neurone 1 to 2.

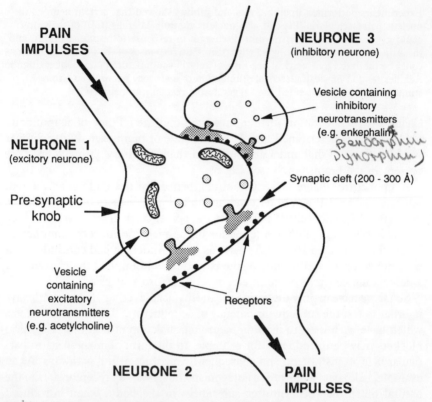

Fig 4.1 Schematic representation of pre-synaptic inhibition Neurone 3, the inhibitory neurone, releases inhibitory neurotransmitters, such as enkephalin, which act to suppress the release of the excitatory transmitter from Neurone 1. This results in attenuation of the transmission of the pain impulse from Neurone 1 to Neurone 2.

Much work has also been done on the nature of opiate receptors with the resultant identification of multiple opiate receptors, some of which are specific to particular (groups of) neurotransmitters whilst others are influenced by a broader group of neuropeptides.[65,66] Furthermore, these receptors are differentially distributed throughout the brain and central nervous system yet are ubiquitous in their influence.[67,68]

There are approximately 50 different neurotransmitters which have been identified to date in humans.[53 (p 104)] A large number of these have been determined to be involved in the mediation of the acupuncture effect. The box on page 90 contains a list of the majority of transmitter substances for which research data has positively established some role in acupuncture. The roles of many of these substances will become more explicit in Chapter 5.

It is apparent from the boxed information that many neuronal pathways are affected aside from those that adopt opiate like substances as their transmitters.

For example, in the case of allergic shock reaction, Mu Jian has shown, via the use of chemical antagonists, that the alpha and beta-2 adrenergic receptors are important sites of transmission of the acupuncture influence, an influence which significantly controls the death rate of the experimental animals.[69,70] This suggests there may be a difference between mechanisms underlying the analgesic effect and those permitting a diminished allergic shock reaction.

In the latter case, adrenergic neurones, representing in principle the sympathetic nervous system, are called into action. However, at different times, yet quite significantly, the serotonergic, cholinergic and other pathways are also influenced. Many of these neurotransmitters also behave as hormones. Besides their role in the neurological context, they move about in the cerebrospinal fluid (CSF), and in some cases the bloodstream.

The fact that so many chemical substances have a role to play in maintaining communication between one neurone and another results in a drug vulnerability specifically at the synaptic sites. Introducing drugs that influence these sites is the experimental technique used to assess the importance of specific neurotransmitters during acupuncture. Our earlier example with naloxone illustrates its adoption as an antagonist to opiate neurotransmitters by preferentially taking up receptor sites usually reserved for endorphins and the like. Therefore communications along the original endorphinergic pathways are restricted.

Pomeranz and Mayer were amongst the first to implicate the involvement of endorphins in acupuncture by injection of naloxone.[39,71] Pomeranz's work on mice was soon followed and confirmed by similar experiments in humans[64,72,73], cats[74], rats[75,76], rabbits[73,77], pigs and monkeys[78] and mice.[39]

This produced a windfall of experiments in China and overseas during the late 1970s and early 1980s exploring precisely the role of endorphin and nonendorphin systems in acupuncture anaesthesia and the stereospecificity of the receptors involved. The result of much of this work confirmed the variability and complexity of neurotransmitters and receptors that participate not only in acupuncture anaesthesia, but also acupuncture therapy with any physiological outcome.[79] For example, Pomeranz, at the vanguard in much of this field, illustrated that the neurotransmitter predominantly involved is dependent upon the frequency of stimulation in the case of electroacupuncture.[80] These findings validated earlier work performed in various countries throughout the world,[39,64,74,80] including the studies by Meg Patterson on the treatment of drug addiction.[81] Pomeranz showed that acupuncture anaesthesia due to low frequency stimulation (4Hz) could be completely blocked by naloxone, however naloxone would have no inhibitory effect on acupuncture anaesthesia due to high frequency stimulation (200Hz). Conversely, parachlorophenylalanine, which is a serotonin synthesis inhibitor, reduces high frequency analgesia but produces no effect on low frequency electroacupuncture analgesia. Hence, it seems that electroacupuncture analgesia induced by low frequency stimulation is mediated by endorphins while high frequency stimulation is not endorphinergic but at least partly serotonergic.

Higher low freqs.

Common neurotransmitters involved in acupuncture

Neurotransmitter   Major area of Influence

Neuropeptides (opiate-like substances)

Endorphins
: Each a different fraction of the lipoprotein/ lipotropin substrate. Are found principally in the spinal cord and brain although are also present in the bloodstream. Alpha & beta-endorphins are found particularly in the pituitary.[67] Beta-endorphins are found in the hypothalamus (especially) and rostral brain stem.[97] Endorphins are 4 times more prevalent in the thalamus and hypothalamus than enkephalins and hence may have a more significant role to play in pain management with acupuncture.[68] They are released after stress or painful stimuli.[98] and are closely involved with emotional states.

Enkephalins (leu-enkephalin met-enkephalin)
: Also responsible for presynaptic inhibition in brain. Highest concentrations in the globus pallidus, midbrain, PAG, hypothalamus and limbic areas. Are also found in the dorsal horns in small interneurons. Widely spread in low concentration in the central nervous system, but are rapidly inactivated by endorphins.[67]

Dynorphin A
Dynorphin B
: Dynorphin A and dynorphin B both operate as opioid peptides in the spinal cord.[27,110] Dynorphin B in the spinal cord of the rat may be important in mediating electroacupuncture analgesia.[107]

Substance P
: Is present in substantia gelatinosa in spinal cord, and in brain. Its presence appears to inhibit acupuncture analgesia, however under other conditions it appears to have dual action.[99] Experiments indicate that it many have an analgesic effect in the brain whilst promoting the pain stimulus in the spinal cord.[100,23(p 262),101,102]

Serotonin (5HT)
: Is an inhibitory neurotransmitter which acts particularly in the raphe nuclei and thalamus.[104] Concerned with functions such as pain, sleep, mood-elevation, aggression, appetite. Diminished serotonin levels have been associated with chronic depression and suicidal tendencies.[81 (p 264, p 146)]

Neurotransmitter	Major area of Influence
Simple amino acids Histamine	Content of histamine is highest in skin, lung and peripheral nervous tissue, but also exists in the brain. Its presence in the periphery appears to encourage the pain stimulus whilst in the brain it may play a role similar to morphine.[103]
Bradykinin Cholecystokinin (CCK)	Exists in brain and gut, and in substantia geletinosa of spinal cord. Behaves as an endogenous anti-opiate, and acts to suppress acupuncture analgesia.
Catecholamines Adrenalin (epinephrine) noradrenalin (nor-epin)	Both are secreted by the medullary part of the adrenal gland and found throughout the brain and spinal cord.[67,81] (p 262) Noradrenalin is also found in the N, habenula and the PAG. Noradrenalin in the brain is antagonistic to acupuncture analgesia, whilst in the spinal cord it mediates acupuncture analgesia.[69,70] Central noradrenalin exerts an antagonistic effect on AA via alpha-receptors and an augmentary effect via beta-receptors.[116]
Dopamine	It is found in significant concentration in the basal nuclei of the brain. In inhibits the extrapyramidal system and inhibits acupuncture analgesia.[81] (p 259),116
Acetylcholine *(ACh)*	Predominantly in the parasympathetic nervous system and behaves as an excitatory neurotransmitter. Acetylcholine is an important mediator of AA.[111,116]
Other non-opiates Somatostatin	Is released from the hypothalamus and prevents growth hormone release from the pituitary.
Luteinising hormone releaing hormone (LHRH)	
Thyrotropin-releasing hormone	
Gamma-amino-butyric acid (GABA)	Exists in many areas especially the spinal cord, cerebellum and cortex, with highest concentrations in the midbrain and thalamus.[23] (p 242) It functions as an inhibitory neurotransmitter in all regions of the brain and spinal cord. It may

Neurotransmitter	Major area of Influence
	be related to anxiety states, and is deficient in several neuromuscular diseases.[81] (p 260) It is interesting that it appears to operate antagonistically to acupuncture analgesia.[108,112]
Adrenocorticotrophic hormone (ACTH)	
	Secreted by the pituitary gland to maintain homeostasis in many body functions. Triggers increased release of cortisol when under stress. Increased plasma levels noted under acupuncture.[15,14,115]
Glycine	Inhibits at the spinal cord level.
Glutamic acid	Causes excitation in many regions including the thalamus, limbic system (hippocampus) and cortex.
Prostaglandins	Prostaglandins and enkephalins are mutually antagonistic in context of pain perception.[85]
Cyclic AMP	Intraventricular injections antagonise acupuncture analgesia in rats.[105] Plasma cAMP increases during strong intensity electroacupuncture.[37]
Cyclic GMP	Observed to rise in rat diencephalon and lower brainstem in acupuncture analgesia.[106] In some clinical situations. cGMP is markedly elevated after acupuncture.[109]

This has important implications for treatment with electroacupuncture, in particular choosing which frequency of stimulation to use. For example, serotonin has many physiological properties other than pain relief, including inhibition of gastric secretion (important in the management of stomach ulcers), stimulation of smooth muscles, and the production of vasoconstriction (useful in the management of migraines). Therefore high frequency electroacupuncture may be preferred in illnesses where such factors are important.

Conversely, stimulation frequencies to release endorphins may be more appropriate in acute pain and opiate drug dependencies. The widespread distribution of opiate receptors in the nervous system implies that opiate peptides are involved in a broad range of functions other than analgesia. The endogenous opiates act on prolactin and growth hormone release[82] and are also involved in the inhibition of gastrointestinal motility.[65] Morphine itself is known to cause sleepiness, mood changes and alterations of activity levels.

This kind of data is important to bear in mind when reviewing the work of prominent physicians and authors on acupuncture, such as Dr Julian Kenyon.[83] Contrary to an enormous wealth of information in this area, his trial on naloxone intervention in the acupuncture treatment of chronic pain concludes that the hypothesis that acupuncture therapy is mediated even in part by endorphins cannot be supported. Although Kenyon does not use electroacupuncture, in his report he makes no mention of the needle technique adopted or the points needled (Yet both factors have been well established as important criteria affecting the outcome of acupuncture, reported by the Chinese from the earliests texts, and confirmed scientifically more recently—see Ch. 3.)

Other suggestions have been made that, whilst low frequency stimulation is mediated by endorphins, high frequency stimulation is strictly segmental and interferes with the transmission in the pain pathway in the central nervous system at the segmental level.[84]

Antagonist drugs which block the nerve impulse are not the only chemical substances which are introduced experimentally to assess the significance of particular neurotransmitters. Drugs which increase the synthesis or degradation of neurotransmitters may also be employed during acupuncture to witness amelioration or deterioration of response, and thereby determine the importance of any particular neurotransmitter.

Prevention of the degradation of endorphins will prolong and promote electroacupuncture anaesthesia. This has been demonstrated by Pomeranz with the application of D-amino acids (DAA).[74] DAA blocks the peptidases, e.g., carboxypeptidase A, which normally breaks down peptides such as endorphins. Introduction of DAA will increase the electroacupuncture analgesia effect by increasing available endorphin, a consequence of its decreased rate of destruction. Naloxone, of course, may still be used to block this rise in analgesia.[85,86]

The drug reserpine, on the other hand, releases serotonin from the presynaptic terminals of the descending monoaminergic tracts, and by doing so enhances the analgesic effect of acupuncture at least in rabbits, despite the fact that it blocks morphine analgesia. The monoaminergic tracts terminate in the dorsal horns, but serotonin may also transfuse through the cerebrospinal fluid to various spinal levels and in this fashion also exert a blocking influence on ascending pain impulses. Of course, diffusion through the cerebrospinal fluid would be considerably slower than any direct neural transmission.

Accumulation of these research results detailing responses to nerve sections and chemical nerve agonists and antagonists strongly underscores the importance of the neural mediation of the acupuncture effect. However, caution is needed here not to make too much of a quantum leap by assuming that nerves mark the beginning and end of acupuncture therapy.

It is worthwhile at this stage to contrast our neural paradigm with the sort of research which highlights the humoral responses to acupuncture.

Humoral mediation

Many biochemical substances which behave as neurotransmitters exhibit an humoral nature. All do at least in the context of the cerebrospinal fluid, but some others pass through the blood-brain barrier and hence circulate in the bloodstream.[23 (p 213),55]

That humoral factors are active in acupuncture is shown by many of the characteristics of therapy. In acupuncture analgesia, for example, it takes approximately 20 minutes for the analgesia to be established, and then diminished pain sensation may last for up to an hour after the needles are removed.[63,74]

The treatment of some diseases such as psoriasis and other skin disorders, menstrual disorders, and viral or bacterial infections would be more easily explained if humoral factors were taken into consideration. I have already shown that blood cell, hormone and immune factors change with treatment, but this does not necessarily mean they are primary mechanisms of acupuncture. However, there are some experiments designed to assess the importance of these humoral factors as mediators of the physiological changes due to needling. For example, in China and elsewhere, many experiments have been performed on rabbits,[87] dogs, cats, oxen and rats,[88] where blood is circulated between an acupunctured animal and an unneedled partner. The same, albeit diminished, acupuncture effect is observed in the unneedled partner.

Similarly, exchange of cerebrospinal fluid (CSF) between experimental animals by aspiration from the lateral ventricles, results in the same acupuncture analgesic effect in the unneedled partner, thereby also lending support to the argument that humoral factors operate as an integral part of acupuncture. In 1974 Chinese workers in Beijing transfered CSF from acupunctured mice to observe raised analgesia levels in the recipient, unacupunctured mice.[89] This result was more clearly understood after Sjolund and fellow workers in Sweden identified the increased presence of endorphins in the CSF of human patients after electroacupuncture.[90] Zhang Anzhong[37] also describes related Chinese experimental findings where cerebrospinal fluid was removed from the lateral ventricles after acupuncture in humans and increased endorphin activity observed,[91] and from rabbits, with higher enkephalin contents noted.[92] Further, in 1980 Clement-Jones and colleagues found increased beta-endorphins, but not met-enkephalins in human CSF after acupuncture.[93]

Increased serotonin content in the cerebrospinal fluid could also explain the effects of these CSF exchanges. However, whilst the endorphins and enkephalins pass the bloodbrain barrier to some extent[23 (p 243),72] serotonin does not normally permeate it, and its increased presence in the bloodstream after acupuncture may be the result of some precurser, such as tryptophan, initially entering the bloodstream or the direct release of serotonin by the pituitary.

Many experiments have measured increases in neurohumoral factors in the bloodstream.[72] For example, Nappi and colleagues state that the plasma level of beta-endorphin, beta-lipotropin and ACTH are all increased under acupuncture.[15] These substances may in turn exert an influence on other tissues and glands. Raised ACTH plasma levels as a consequence of stimulation of the pituitary by acupuncture could be responsible for an increase of corticosteroids from the adrenal cortex, and result in the inhibition of inflammatory reactions observed in, say, the treatment of acute or chronic arthritis.[94,95]

Finally, opiates are also released directly from the pituitary into the blood-stream and give added credibility to the raised generalised analgesia levels, however opiates do not explain the specific localised effects so frequently seen in acupuncture analgesia. These localised effects point us once again to the existence of a central biasing system that controls impulse transmission in a selective fashion.[96] And our argument reverts to the simultaneous existence at least of neural transmission in acupuncture.

REFERENCES

1. Mendelson G, Selwood T S, Kranz H, Loh T S, Kidson M A, Scott D S 1983 Acupuncture treatment of chronic back pain: a double-blind placebo-controlled trial. American Journal of Medicine 74: 49–55
2. Chiang C Y, Chang C T, Chu H, Yang L 1973 Peripheral afferent pathway for acupuncture analgesia. Scientia Sinica 16(2): 210–217
3. Eisenberg D 1986 Encounters with Qi. Jonathan Cape, London
4. Takeshige C 1983 The central mechanism of analgesia in acupuncture anaesthesia—differentiation of acupuncture point and non-point by the central analgesia producing system. Acupuncture and Electrotherapeutics Research 8(3/4): 323–324
5. Takeshige C 1985 Differentiation between acupuncture and non-acupuncture points by association with analgesia inhibitory system. Acupuncture and Electrotherapeutics Research 10: 195–203
6. Zhang R, Zhao H 1984 Effect of AQSD resulted from Neiguan needling in cardiovascular disease; analysis of 112 cases. Journal of Traditional Chinese Medicine 4(4): 269–272
7. Meng Z, Zhu Z, Hu X 1984 New development in the researches of meridian phenomena in China during the past five years. Acupuncture Research 9(3): 207–222
8. Lee T N 1978 Thalamic neurone theory and classical acupuncture. American Journal of Acupuncture 6: 273–282
9. Jayasuriya A, Fernando F 1978 The motor gate theory: neurophysiological model to explain the phenomenon of late motor recovery following use of acupuncture in paralytic conditions. American Journal of Acupuncture 6: 197–204
10. Shen A C, Whitehouse M J, Powers T R, Young R C, Engleman E P 1973 A pilot study of the effects of acupuncture in rheumatoid arthritis. Arthritis and Rheumatism 16: 569–570 16: 569–570
11. Wientraub M, Petursson S, Schwartz M et al 1975 Acupuncture in musculoskeletal pain: methodology and results in a double-blind controlled clinical trial. Clinical Pharmacology and Therapeutics 17: 248
12. Man S C, Baragar F D 1973 Preliminary clinical study of acupuncture in rheumatoid arthritis with painful knees. Arthritis and Rheumatism 16(4): 558–559
13. Knox V J, Handfield-Jones C E, Shum K 1979 Subject expectancy and the reduction of cold pressor pain with acupuncture and placebo acupuncture. Psychosomatic Medicine 41(6): 477–486
14. Meyer F P, Nebrensky A 1983 A double-blind comparative study of micro-stimulation and placebo effect in short term treatment of the chronic back pain patient. California Health Review 2(1) Aug/Sept
15. Nappi G, Facchinetti F, Legnante G et al 1982 Different releasing effects of traditional manual acupuncture and electroacupuncture on propriocortin-related peptides. Acupuncture and Electrotherapeutics Research 7: 93–103
16. Fung K P, Chow O K W, So S Y 1986 Attenuation of exercise induced asthma by acupuncture. Lancet Dec. 20/27: 1419–1421
17. MacDonald A J R, Macrae K D, Master B R, Rubin A P 1983 Superficial acupuncture in the relief of chronic low back pain: a placebo controlled randomised trial. Annals of the Royal College of Surgeons England 65: 44–46

18. Peng A T C, Behar S, Yue S J 1987 Long term therapeutic effects of EA for chronic neck and shoulder pain: a double blind study. Acupuncture and Electrotherapeutics Research 12(1): 37–44
19. Shibutani K, Kubal K 1979 Similarities of prolonged pain relief produced by nerve block and acupuncture in patients with chronic pain. Acupuncture and Electrotherapeutics Research 4: 9–16
20. Kaptchuk T 1983 The web that has no weaver: understanding Chinese medicine. Rider, London
21. Karczyn A D 1978 Mechanism of placebo analgesia. Lancet 2: 1304–1305
22. Levine J D, Gordon N C, Fields H L 1978 The mechanism of placebo analgesia. Lancet 2: 654–657
23. Needham J, Lu G D 1980 Celestial lancets: a history and rationale of acupuncture and moxibustion. Cambridge University Press, Cambridge
24. Knox V J, Shum K 1977 Reduction of cold pressor pain with acupuncture analgesia in high and low hypnotic subjects. Journal of Abnormal Psychology 86: 639–643
25. Levy B, Matsumoto T 1975 Pathophysiology of acupuncture: nervous system transmission. American Journal of Surgery June p378–384
26. PLA Veterinary Diseases Prevention Research Institute 1979 The application of acupuncture anaesthesia in operations of domestic animals. National Symposium of Acupuncture and Moxibustion and Acupuncture Anaesthesia, Beijing Paper No 200
27. Han J 1984 On the mechanisms of acupuncture analgesia. Acupuncture Research 9(3): 237–245
28. Beijing Childrens' Hospital 1975 A clinical analysis of 1474 operations under AA among children. Chinese Medical Journal 1(5): 369–374
29. Xu L, Fu Z, Xiang M et al 1979 The effect of acupuncture analgesia and its relation to blood endorphin, blood histamine and suggestibility. National Symposium of Acupuncture and Moxibustion and Acupuncture Anaesthesia, Beijing Paper No 510
30. Vidal C, Jacob J 1986 Hyperalgesia induced by emotional stress in the rat: an experimental model of human anxiogenic hyperalgesia. Annals of the New York Academy of Science 467: 73–81
31. Kelly D D, Bodnar R J 1979 Intrinsic non-opiate mechanisms of analgesia. Letter to Acupuncture and Electrotherapeutics Research 4: 159–161
32. Kelly D D (ed) 1986 Stress-induced analgesia. Annals of the New York Academy of Sciences vol 467
33. Eriksson M B E, Sjolund B H, Nielzen S 1979 Long term results of peripheral conditioning stimulation as an analgesic measure of chronic pain. Pain 6: 335–347
34. Sjolund B H, Eriksson M 1979 The influence of naloxone on analgesia produced by peripheral conditioning stimulation. Brain Research 173: 295–301
35. Watkins L R, Mayer D J 1986 Multiple endogenous opiate and non-opiate analgesia systems: evidence of their existence and clinical implications. Annals of the New York Academy of Science 467: 273–299
36. Curzon G, Hutson P H, Kennet G A, Marcou M, Gower A, Tricklebank M D 1986 Characteristics of analgesias induced by brief or prolonged stress. Annals of the New York Academy of Sciences 467: 93–103
37. Zhang A Z 1980 Endorphin and acupuncture analgesia research in the People's Republic of China (1975–1979). Acupuncture and Electrotherapeutics Research 5: 131–146
38. Pomeranz B 1986 Relation of stress-induced analgesia to acupuncture analgesia. Annals of the New York Academy of Science 467: 444–447
39. Pomeranz B H, Chiu D 1976 Naloxone blockade of acupuncture analgesia: endorphin implicated. Life Sciences 19: 1757–1762
40. Chapman C R, Wilson M E, Gehrig J D 1976 Comparative effects of acupuncture and transcutaneous stimulation on the perception of painful dental stimuli. Pain 2: 265–283
41. Peets J M, Pomeranz B 1985 Acupuncture-like transcutaneous electrical wave stimulation analgesia is influenced by spinal cord endorphins but not serotonin: an intrathecal pharmacological study. In: Advances in Pain Research and Therapy. 9: Raven Press, New York 519–52
42. Cheng R, Pomeranz B 1981 Monoaminergic mechanism of electroacupuncture analgesia. Brain Research 215: 77–92
43. Cheng R, McKibbin L, Roy B, Pomeranz B 1980 International Journal of Neuroscience 10: 95–97

44. Shanghai College of Traditional Chinese Medicine 1981 Acupuncture; a comprehensive text O'Connor J, Bensky D (trans) Eastland Press, Seattle
45. Zhang A, Xu S, Zeng D, Zhang L 1979 The effects of naloxone on acupuncture analgesia produced by different strength of electric stimulation. National Symposium of Acupuncture and Moxibustion and Acupuncture Anaesthesia, Beijing Paper No 496
46. Zborowski M 1952 Cultural components in response to pain. Journal of Social Issues 8: 16
47. Josey C, Miller C 1932 Race, sex and class differences in the ability to endure pain. Journal of Social Psychology 3: 364
48. Kaptchuk T, Croucher M 1986 The healing arts. British Broadcasting Corporation, London
49. Kleinman A 1980 Patients and healers in the context of culture. University of California Press, Berkeley
50. Wang J Y 1983 Psychosomatic illness in the Chinese cultural context. In Romanucci-Ross L, The anthropology of medicine; from culture to method. Bergin & Garvey Massachusetts
51. Peets J M, Pomeranz B 1978 CXBK mice deficient in opiate receptors show poor electro-acupuncture analgesia. Nature 273: 675–676
52. Jacob J J, Nicola M A, Michaud G, Vidal C, Prudhomme N 1986 Genetic modulations of stress-induced analgesia in mice. Annals of the New York Academy of Sciences 467: 104–115
53. Bergland R 1985 The fabric of mind. Penguin, Melbourne
54. Lee D C 1974 Cardiovascular effects of acupuncture in anesthetized dogs. American Journal of Chinese Medicine 2(3): 271–282
55. Omura Y 1975 Pathophysiology of acupuncture treatment: effects of acupuncture on cardiovascular and nervous systems. Acupuncture and Electrotherapeutics Research 1: 51–140
56. MacDonald A J R 1983 Segmental acupuncture therapy. Acupuncture and Electrotherapeutics Research. 8: 267–282
57. Mu J 1985 Nanjing College of Traditional Chinese Medicine, Personal communication
58. Mu J 1984 Paper presented at the Fourth Advanced Acupuncture Studies Course, Nanjing
59. Bossy J 1984 Morphological data concerning the acupuncture points and channel network. Acupuncture and Electrotherapeutics Research 9: 79–106
60. Chiang C Y, Liu J I, Chu T H, Pai Y H, Chang S C 1975 Studies on the spinal ascending pathway for the effect of acupuncture analgesia in rabbits. Scientia Sinica 18(5): 651
61. Chang H T 1973 Integrative action of the thalamus in the process of acupuncture for analgesia. Scientia Sinica 16(1): 25
62. Shen E, Tshai T T, Lan C 1975 Supraspinal participation in the inhibitory effect of acupuncture on viscero-somatic reflex discharges. Chinese Medical Journal 1: 431
63. Anderson S A, Ericson T, Holmgren E, Lindqvist G 1973 Electroacupuncture effect on pain threshold measured with electrical stimulation of teeth. Brain Research 63: 393–396
64. Mayer D J, Price D D, Rafii A 1977 Antagonism of acupuncture analgesia in man by the narcotic naloxone. Brain Research 121: 368–372
65. Pasternak G W 1986 Multiple morphine and enkephalin receptors: biochemical and pharmacological aspects. Annals of the New York Academy of Science 467: 130–139
66. Cheng R, Pomeranz B 1980 Electroacupuncture analgesia is mediated by stereospecific opiate receptors and is reversed by antagonists of type 1 receptors. Life Sciences 26: 631–638
67. Lord J A H, Waterfield A A, Hughes J, Kosterlitz H W 1977 Endogenous opioid peptides: multiple agonists and receptors. Nature 267: 495–497
68. Chang K J, Cooper B R, Hazum E, Cuatrecasas P 1979 Multiple opiate receptors: different regional distribution in the brain and differential binding of opiates and opioid peptides. Molecular Pharmacology 16: 91–104
69. Mu J 1985 Influence of adrenergic antagonist and naloxone on the anti-allergic effect of electroacupuncture in mice. Acupuncture and Electrotherapeutics Research 10: 163–167
70. Mu J 1982 Effect of acupuncture on allergic shock of experimental mice. Shanghai Journal of Acupuncture and Moxibustion 3: 195–197
71. Mayer D J, 1975 Pain inhibition by electrical brain stimulation: comparison to morphine. Neurosciences Research Program Bulletin 13: 94–100
72. Malizia E, Andreucci G, Paolucci D, Crescenzi F, Fabbri A, Fraioli F 1979 Electroacupuncture and peripheral beta-endorphin and ACTH levels. Lancet 2: 535–536

73. He L F, Dong W Q 1983 Activity of opioid peptidergic system in acupuncture analgesia. Acupuncture and Electrotherapeutics Research 8: 257–266
74. Pomeranz B, Cheng R 1979 Suppression of noxious responses in single neurons of cat spinal cord by electroacupuncture and its reversal by the opiate antagonist naloxone. Experimental Neurology 64(2): 327–341
75. Takeshige C, Luo P C, Kamada Y, Oka K, Murai M, Hisamitsu T 1978 Relationship between midbrain neurones (periaquaductal grey and midbrain reticular formation) and acupuncture analgesia, animal hypnosis. In: Bonica JJ (ed) Advances in Pain Research and Therapy 3: 615–621. Raven Press, New York
76. Takeshige C, Sato K, Komugi H 1980 Role of periaquaductal central grey in AA. Acupuncture and Electrotherapeutics Research 5: 323–337
77. Zhou G Z, Xu S F, Zhang A Z 1980 The effect of naloxone on electroacupuncture analgesia in rabbits. Acupuncture and Electrotherapeutics Research 5(2): 197–199
78. Huang Y, Wang Q W, Zheng J Z, Li D R, Xie G Y 1986 Analgesic effects of several modes of electroacupuncture in monkeys and their reversal by naloxone. In: Zhang X T (ed) Research on acupuncture, moxibustion and acupuncture anesthesia. Science Press, Beijing
79. Pasternak G W 1981 Central mechanisms of opioid analgesia. Acupuncture and Electrotherapeutics Research 6: 135–149
80. Pomeranz B, Cheng R S S 1979 Electroacupuncture analgesia could be mediated by at least two pain-relieving mechanisms; endorphin and non-endorphin systems. Life Sciences 25: 1957–1962
81. Patterson M 1986 Hooked? NET: the new approach to drug cure. Faber and Faber, London
82. Bloom F, Segal D, Ling N, Guillemin R 1976 Endorphins: profound behavioural effects in rats suggest new etiological factors in mental illness. Science 194: 630–632
83. Kenyon J N, Knight C J, Wells C 1983 Randomised double-blind trial on the immediate effects of naloxone on classical Chinese acupuncture therapy for chronic pain. Acupuncture and Electrotherapeutics Research 8:17–24
84. Cheng R S S, Pomeranz B 1980 A combined treatment with d-amino acids and electroacupuncture produces a greater analgesia than either treatment alone; naloxone reverses these effects. Pain 8: 231–236
85. Ehrenpreis S, Balagot R C, Comaty J E, Myles S B 1978 Naloxone-reversible analgesia in mice produced by D-phenylananine and hydrocinnamic acid inhibitors of carboxypeptidase-A. In: Bonica JJ (ed) Advances in Pain Research and Therapy 3: 479–486. Raven Press, New York
86. Ehrenpreis S 1983 Potentiation of AA by inhibitors of endorphin degradation. Acupuncture and Electrotherapeutics Research 8: 319–345
87. Yang M M P, Kok S H 1979 Further study of the neurohumoral factor endorphin in the mechanism of AA. American Journal of Chinese Medicine 7(2): 143–148
88. Lung C H, Sun A C, Tsao C J, Chang Y L, Fan L 1974 An observation of the humoral factor in AA in rats. American Journal of Chinese Medicine 2: 203–205
89. Beijing Research Group of Acupuncture Anaesthesia 1974 The role of some neurotransmitters of brain in finger acupuncture analgesia. Scientia Sinica 17: 112–130
90. Sjolund B, Terenius L, Eriksson M 1977 Increased CSF levels of endorphins after electroacupuncture. Acta Physiologica Scandinavia 100: 382–384
91. Pan X P, Lou X H, Yao S Y et al 1979 The relationship between the human CSF levels of endorphins and acupuncture analgesia. National Symposium of Acupuncture and Moxibustion and Acupuncture Anaesthesia, Beijing Paper No 494
92. Zou G, Wu S X, Wang F S et al 1979 Increased levels of endorphins in the cisternal cerebrospinal fluid of rabbits in acupuncture analgesia. National Symposium of Acupuncture and Moxibustion and Acupuncture Anaesthesia, Beijing Paper No 491
93. Clement-Jones V, Tomlin S, Rees L H, McLoughlin L, Besser G M, Wen H L 1980 Increased beta-endorphin but not met-enkephalin levels in human CSF after acupuncture for recurrent pain. Lancet 2: 946–948
94. Wen W L, Ho W K K, Wong H K, Mehal Z D, Ng Y H, Ma L 1978 Reductions of adrenocorticotropic hormone (ACTH) and cortisol in drug addicts treated by acupuncture and electrical stimulation (AES). Chinese Medicine: East & West 6(1): 61–66
95. Wen W L, Ho W K K, Wong H K, Mehal Z D, Ng Y H, Ma L 1978 Changes in

adrenocorticotropic hormone (ACTH) and cortisol levels in drug addicts treated by a new and rapid detoxification procedure using acupuncture and naloxone. Chinese Medicine: East & West 6(3): 241–246

96. Oliveras J L, Besson J M, Guilbaud G, Liebeskind J C 1974 Behavioural and electrophysiological evidence of pain inhibition from midbrain stimulation in the cat. Experimental Brain Research 20: 32–44
97. Abrams G M, Recht L 1982 Neuropeptides and their role in pain and analgesia. Acupuncture and Electrotherapeutics Research 7: 105–121
98. Guillemin R, Vargo T, Rossier J et al 1977 Beta-endorphin and adrenocorticotrophin are secreted concomitantly by the pituitary gland. Science 197: 1367–1368
99. Zhang C L, Sun G D, Yan H J et al 1986 Substance P: its analgesic effect and influence on caudate neuronal activity in conscious rabbits. In: Zhang X T (ed) 1986 Research on acupuncture, moxibustion, and acupuncture anaesthesia. Science Press, Beijing, p388–396
100. Frederickson R C A, Burgis V, Harrell C E, Edwards J D 1978 Dual actions of substance P on nociception: possible role of endogenous opioids. Science 199: 1359–1362
101. Oehme P, Hilse H, Morgenstern E, Gores E 1980 Substance P: does it produce analgesia or hyperalgesia? Science 208: 305–307
102. Randic M, Miletic V 1977 Effect of substance P in cat dorsal horn neurones activated by noxious stimuli. Brain Research 128: 164
103. Lu Z S, Cheng J 1986 Role of histamine in acupuncture analgesia. In Zhang X T (ed) 1986 Research on acupuncture, moxibustion, and acupuncture anaesthesia. Science Press, Beijing
104. Wang Y J, Wang S K 1987 The role of alpha and beta receptors and their regulation of 5-HT metabolism of rat brain in electroacupuncture analgesia. Journal of Traditional Chinese Medicine 7(1): 57–62
105. Qiu X C, Gia G L, Han C S 1979 Effect of intraventricular injection of cAMP on acupuncture analgesia and mophine analgesia in rats. Journal of the Peking Medical College, 1: 4–6
106. Lu Z S 1983 The relationship between cAMP and cGMP in regions of rat brain and acupuncture analgesia. Journal of Traditional Chinese Medicine 3(1): 3–6
107. Xie G X, Han J S 1984 Dynorphin-B (Rimorphin) mediates electroacupuncture analgesia in the spinal cord of the rat. Second National Symposium on Acupuncture and Moxibustion and Acupuncture Anaesthesia, Beijing Paper No 446
108. Fan S G, Qu Z C, Zhai Q Z, Han J S 1984 Cerebral GABA: antagonistic effects on electroacupuncture analgesia and morphine analgesia in rats. Second National Symposium on Acupuncture and Moxibustion and Acupuncture Anaesthesia, Beijing Paper No. 491
109. Li C J, Bi L G, Zhu B J et al 1986 Effects of acupuncture on left ventricular function, microcirculation, cAMP and cGMP of acute myocardial infarction patients. Journal of Traditional Chinese Medicine 6(3): 157–161
110. Han J S, Xie G X, Xie C W 1984 Dynorphin has a potent analgesic action and mediates electroacupuncture analgesia in the spinal cord of the rabbit. Second National Symposium on Acupuncture and Moxibustion and Acupuncture Anaesthesia, Beijing Paper No. 445
111. Guan X M, Yu B, Wang C Y, Liu X C, 1986 The role of cholinergic nerves in electroacupuncture analgesia - influence of acetylcholine, eserine, neostigmine, and hemicholinum on electroacupuncture analgesia. In: Zhang X T (ed) Research on acupuncture, moxibustion, and acupuncture anaesthesia. Science Press, Beijing
112. Meng J B, Fu W X, Cai J H, Qi Y Z Yao S Z 1986 Effect of electroacupuncture on the oxygen metabolism of myocardium during myocardial ischaemic injury. Journal of Traditional Chinese Medicine 6(2): 201–206
113. Mann F 1983 Scientific aspects of acupuncture. Heinemann, London
114. Omura Y 1976 Pathophysiology of acupuncture effects, ACTH, morphine-like substances, pain, phantom pain and itch, brain microcirculation, and memory. Acupuncture and Electrotherapeutics Research 2: 1–32
115. Omura Y 1978 Pain threshold measurement before and after acupuncture: contraversial results of radiant heat method and electrical method, and the roles of ACTH-like substances and endorphins. Acupuncture and Electrotherapeutics Research 3: 1–21
116. Han J S, Tang J, Ren M F, Zhou Z F, Fan S G, Qui X S 1980 Central neurotransmitters and acupuncture analgesia. American Journal of Chinese Medicine 8(4): 331–348

FURTHER READING

Akil H 1975 Opiates; biological mechanisms. In: Barcas J D (ed) Psychopharmacology; from theory to practice. Oxford University Press, New York p 292–305
Basbaum A I, Fields H L 1984 Endogenous pain control systems: brainstem spinal pathways and endorphin circuitry. Annual Review of Neuroscience 7: 309–338
Goldstein A, Hilgard E R 1975 Failure of the opiate antagonist naloxone to modify hypnotic analgesia. Proceedings National Academy of Science 72: 2041–2045
Kronger WS 1960 Hypnoanaesthesia in surgery and obstetrics. Western Journal of Surgery Obstetrics and Gynecology 68: 72–75
Lee D C 1975 Cardiovascular effects of moxibustion at Renzhong (Du 26) during halothane anesthesia in dogs. American Journal of Chinese Medicine (3): 245–260.
Romanucci-Ross L et al 1983 The anthropology of medicine; from culture to method. Bergin and Garvey Publ., Massachusetts
Small T J 1974 The neurophysiological basis for acupuncture. American Journal of Acupuncture 2(2): 77–87
Steiner R P 1983 Acupuncture—cultural perspectives. Postgraduate Medicine 74(4): 60–66
Watkins L R, Mayer D J 1982 Organisation of endogenous opiate and non-opite pain control system. Science 216: 1185–1192

5. The role of the central nervous system in acupuncture

So far we have discussed only in general terms the neurological changes under acupuncture. In this chapter we will look at some specific sites where neurological interactions occur and explore some of the theories proposed to explain the actions of acupuncture.

It should be reemphasised here that it is not my intent to justify acupuncture in western scientific terms. To the traditionally trained doctor in TCM there is already an elaborate theory that permits the careful prescription of acupuncture points as treatment. Observations of neurological interactions give little assistance in the actual management of illness, in that they do not support old or create new theoretical models and guidance how best to manage disease with acupuncture. This contrasts sharply with the Chinese theories which do act as guidelines to appropriate treatment.

Nevertheless, it is worthwhile focusing on some of the more detailed work on the neurological interactions of acupuncture and any theories that may emanate from this research. The work in itself appears capable of expanding the spectrum of applications for acupuncture, such as the management of drug withdrawal, the use of acupuncture for analgesia in surgery, or any other non-traditional applications. Increasing biomedical understanding of acupuncture also encourages the development of techniques such as scalp acupuncture.

The role of the central nervous system in acupuncture is outlined in this chapter by discussing the most important sites in the central nervous system where acupuncture is known to wield major influence. This is only an outline and the research is much more extensive than reported here. For each relevant brain region the chapter reviews the neurotransmitters of significance in acupuncture, however most neurotransmitters are found to some degree in any brain region, where they may also play a relatively major role. The reader should bear in mind that the following accounts are certainly not a definitive statement of the workings of acupuncture in the central nervous system.

INTERACTION AT THE LEVEL OF THE SPINAL CORD

The spinothalamic tract, running from the spinal level to the brain, is the principal nerve tract responsible for the transmission of pain signals. It would appear logical that attenuation of pain signals could occur if acupuncture influenced the key locations of this tract, namely the synapses at the spinal level and thalamus in the lower brain (see Fig. 5.1). These two regions of the central nervous system have been subjected to a great deal of investigation in the search for an explanation of how acupuncture might alter the pattern of neurological behaviour at these sites. To commence with I will outline the main outcomes of such work at the spinal cord level.

For a while the best established theory to explain the anodyne effects of acupuncture was the gate control mechanism, which was conceived initially to operate at the spinal cord level. Later research has certainly eclipsed its value as a theoretical model, although it may have assisted to answer some western medical queries on the mechanics of acupuncture.

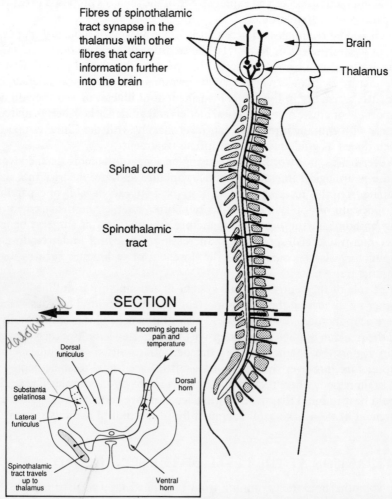

Fig. 5.1 Spinothalamic tract with principal synaptic locations at the spinal cord level in the substantia gelatinosa and at the thalamus.

The gate control theory proposes that pain signals and the acupuncture stimulus travel on different sized nerve fibres and interact at specific sites to inhibit competitively the painful impulses from being registered higher in the brain. Melzack and Wall in 1965 were the first to propose this gate control mechanism, with their functional gate located in the substantia gelatinosa of the dorsal horns of the spinal cord (see Fig. 5.1).[1] This was endorsed later, in 1973, by the Shenyang Medical College,[2] and reviewed and confirmed in 1978 by Wall.[3]

In order to understand how this inhibition of pain signals occurs, we need to be equipped with some knowledge of the classification of nerve fibre types. The larger, rapidly conducting myelinated nerves are the A-fibres and it is precisely these fibres, particularly the A-beta type, that were thought by Melzack and others[4,5,6] to be the carriers of stimuli such as the pinpricks of acupuncture. The thin, slowly conducting, less or unmyelinated fibres, on the other hand (in this case the A-delta and C fibres) are commonly thought to be the carriers of the pain stimulus (Fig. 5.2). At the site of the substantia gelatinosa in the dorsal horns, Melzack and Wall proposed that a jamming of the pain signals on the thin, slow fibres occurs by the rapid arrival of volleys of impulses transmitted by the larger, myelinated fibres.[1]

Melzack and Wall also proposed that this jamming occurs as a result of presynaptic inhibition of the pain signals, although they did not rule out the possibility of postsynaptic inhibition, or even the presence of descending control from higher level brain centres. In the case of presynaptic inhibition there is a reduction in the amount of transmitter substance secreted at the presynaptic terminal and normally passed on to the next cell. In postsynaptic inhibition the excitability and therefore the response of the postsynaptic neurone terminal is significantly reduced. Nowadays there is ample evidence that both pre-and postsynaptic inhibition occur ubiquitously in acupuncture, and this is supported by what is currently known about the roles of transmitter substances, and by other experiments that monitor the attenuation of cephalic impulses under acupuncture analgesia.

Melzack and Wall's theory also incorporated the possibility that there exists a descending modulation of pain signals by control systems in the brain. However, in the main, their theory discussed how various types of afferent impulses (including acupuncture) could interact and inhibit noxious signals, and also how these inhibitory effects were limited to the spinal segments and their related dermatomes. Their theory implied that the acupuncture stimulus had to be at roughly the same spinal level as the incoming pain signals in order for the two to interact therapeutically at any dorsal horn synapse. The theory was widely adopted in the West although it ignored the complexity of acupuncture that TCM was familiar with.

For example, points such as Renzhong (Du 26) and Houxi (SI 3) are commonly used to treat low back pain. Successful use of either of these points could not be readily explained by the gate control theory as it was first proposed. The early version of the theory failed to explain why analgesia works well in areas where the acupuncture stimulus might not have any direct

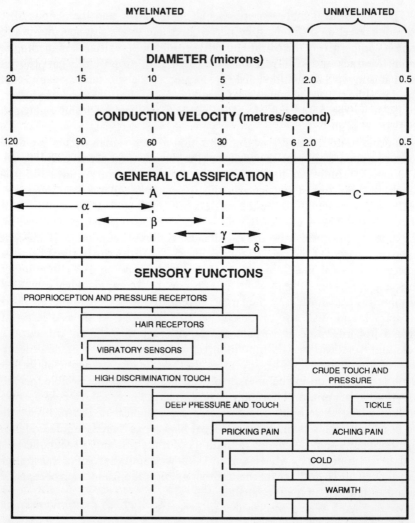

Fig. 5.2 Basic classifications and functions of sensory nerve fibres. (Modified with permission Guyton AC 1982 Human physiology and mechanisms of disease. WB Saunders, Philadelphia, p 365)

segmental input. Furthermore, it could not account for why acupuncture works well in areas supplied by the cranial nerves, where no substantia gelatinosa is present.

Inevitably, medical theorists had to incorporate some concept of neural inhibition at higher centres (such as the thalamus) in order to cater logically for all the possibilities that acupuncture offered. Some years later Man and Chen included the concept of the thalamic gate, and the thalamus has been a focus of research in recent years.[5,6] Man and Chen's revised gate theory, with one gate placed in the thalamus and one still in the spinal cord, was capable of incorporating the influence of the cranial nerves, and thereby making allowance for the fact that acupuncture is able to exert an influence on diseases of the head and face. It also permitted an understanding of how acupuncture is able to exert an influence in regions remote from the dermatomal area of needling. Melzack and Jeans subsequently proposed a simliar two gate theory but placed their second gate in the brainstem.[4]

The levels at which the inhibitory gates were sited, was not to be the only failure of Melzack and Wall's theory when applied to acupuncture. Medical workers in Xian have found that acupuncture sensations travel in both large and small diameter nerve fibres. Han Jisheng, in summarising some of the Chinese research, states that both A-beta and A-delta fibres carry the acupuncture stimulus and inhibit dorsal horn cells of 1st and 5th laminae, which contradicts the gate proposal where the acupuncture signals travel along the large fibres and pain impulses along the thin.[7] Spinal transections performed in Nanjing Medical College demonstrated that the antero-lateral funiculus (namely the spinothalamic tract carrying information of pain and temperature) is the principal afferent pathway of acupuncture analgesia, whilst the dorsal funiculus (lemniscal pathway) is unimportant.[9] However, the spinothalamic tract, which consists of the thinner A-delta and C class fibres, does not carry the acupuncture impulses according to the gate control theory. Like Han Jisheng's claims, these Nanjing experiments again contradict some of the fundamental concepts of the gate control theory.

Melzack's later papers also expanded upon, and gave full recognition to, the role of the reticular formation in the brainstem and other higher level sites such as the cortex, but both in relation to descending modulation of pain signals and not necessarily as inhibitory gates.[8] Some fibres ascending as the anterolateral funiculus of the spinal cord project to the reticular formation (spinoreticular tract), the periaqueductal grey and the intralaminary nuclei of the thalamus (spinothalamic tract). All these structures play an important role in the modulation of pain. From these structures in the brain certain fibres descend to inhibit or facilitate impulse transmission at the spinal cord level. In particular, stemming from the reticular formation and the raphe nuclei in the brainstem, monoamine fibres (that use neurotransmitters containing only one amino acid such as dopamine, noradrenalin, and serotonin) descend and terminate in the substantia gelatinosa of the dorsal horns. This descending inhibitory corridor is the dorsolateral aspect of the spinal cord, transection of which at various levels results in the attenuation of acupuncture analgesia below that level.[9] Hence, the pain and possibly acupuncture signals carried along the anterolateral funiculus to the medial reticular formation in the brainstem, initiate descending impulses along the dorsolateral funiculus that have an inhibiting effect on the transmission of pain signals (Fig. 5.3).

The periaqueductal grey also seems to exert its influence indirectly on the dorsal horn through the nucleus raphe magnus.[10,11] Of the two it is the raphe magnus that is more richly endowed in opiate receptors, permitting it to detect the presence of endogenous opioids, (or morphine), and respond by transmitting messages to the spinal cord, specifically the substantia gelatinosa, via descending serotonergic fibres. At the dorsal horn of the spinal cord,

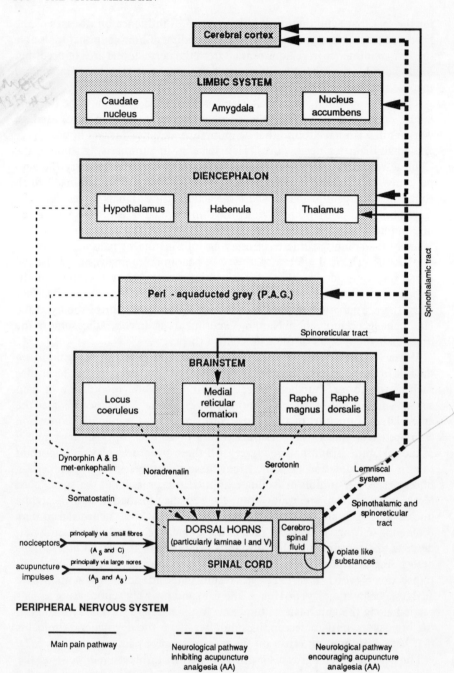

Fig. 5.3 Some of the neurological connections between the brainstem, the spinal cord and peripheral nerves that are activated by acupuncture.

serotonin is released by the terminals of the descending fibres and interferes with the excitatory synaptic processes between the primary pain fibres and the spinal neurones.[12,13,14,15,16,17]

Hence, the acupuncture stimulus (and pain itself), after having risen to regions in the lower brain, may initiate descending impulses along these fibres which travel to the spinal cord synapses, where they help to inhibit or promote the incoming pain signals. Dopamine, noradrenalin, and serotonin may all be released at the spinal level by the descending monoaminergic fibres. These act to attenuate the transmission of painful impulses from the spinal synapses to higher regions in the central nervous system.

Although mostly located in the hypothalamus, some somatostatin neurones are also found in the spinal cord dorsal root where they are assumed to act in a similar way and inhibit pain signals.[18,19] Somatostatin, a peptide hormone and neurotransmitter has been found to behave specifically as a neuronal cell depressant in both the brainstem and dorsal horn of the spinal cord.[20]

In true expression of the yin and yang dichotomy, the inhibitory modulation of pain by acupuncture has its antithesis even at the spinal cord level. Certain substances have been found that encourage the pain signals and help suppress any analgesia brought about by acupuncture. Substance P is one such substance that is involved in pain transmission, particularly in the dorsolateral aspect of the dorsal horns (substance P = Arg-Pro-Lys-Pro-Gln-Gln-Phe-Phe-Gly-Leu-Met NH).[21] Although it exhibits hypotensive and oxytoxic behaviour and is widely distributed in the central and peripheral nervous system, it should be regarded principally as an excitatory transmitter of primary afferent sensory neurons (therefore pain signals). The antagonist lioresal completely inhibits the effects of substance P and by doing so blocks dorsal root transmission.[22,23(p262)] However, substance P when administered peripherally or intraventricularly at certain doses, has been known to produce analgesia, and even be naloxone reversible, implying its association in action with the endogenous opiates.[24,25] Experiments indicate that in the brain it supports the analgesic effect of acupuncture.[123] Its action in conjunction with other neuropeptides is curious, yet, its increased presence in the spinal cord is predominantly inhibitory to acupuncture analgesia.

One other neurotransmitter antagonist to the analgesic effect of acupuncture is cholecystokinin (CCK-8) which, although also found in the dorsal root ganglia, is located more significantly in the cortex, hypothalamus, the limbic system and the periaqueductal grey (PAG) of the brainstem.[21] Amongst the cyclic nucleotides, cAMP also appears to have an antagonistic role in acupuncture and morphine analgesia at spinal sites.[26]

The presence and importance of these neurohumors, highlighted by experiments controlling the analgesic effect of acupuncture, provide strong evidence of the descending inhibitory and excitatory response that acupuncture is capable of initiating. These feedback cycles either complement or oppose the gating mechanism at the spinal cord level.

INTERACTION AT THE LEVEL OF THE BRAINSTEM

The brainstem represents the portion of the brain linking cerebral hemispheres with the spinal cord, and comprises the midbrain, pons and medulla. Due to the significant presence of synapses in this region, the brainstem is an important site for the interference of neural transmission and therefore has a significant role to play in acupuncture analgesia.

Raphe nuclei

The raphe nuclei in the brainstem consists of two principal divisions, the raphe magnus and the raphe dorsalis. It was noted earlier that the terminals of the descending fibres from the periaqueductal grey (PAG) and the raphe nuclei release serotonin and other monoamines in the dorsal horn of the spinal cord.[13,14,15] It appears the PAG exerts its influence indirectly on the dorsal horn through the nucleus raphe magnus.[10,11] These connections from the PAG to the spinal cord via the raphe magnus may represent the main parts of the endogenous analgesic system, and the raphe magnus is presumed to be one of the relay sites in the pathways of descending inhibition.[10,27,28,29]

Zhu Lixia and Shi Qingyao claim that the activation of the raphe magnus, and therefore the descending serotonergic pathway by acupuncture, is partly mediated by opiate like substances from the PAG.[30] (However the PAG is rich not only in opioid peptides but also in opiate receptors).[18,31,32] Acupuncture, focal stimulation of the dorsolateral part of the PAG, and the administration of leucine enkephalin proximal to the raphe magnus neurones could all increase the firing rate of neurones in the raphe magnus. The latter two appear to mimic the effect of acupuncture on the raphe magnus. In any case this increase in spontaneous neuronal discharge in the raphe magnus is blocked by the administration of iontophoretic naloxone. The implication is that acupuncture influences the endogenous analgesic system by encouraging the release of opiates from the PAG and their uptake in the raphe magnus, followed subsequently by the stimulation of the mono-amine tracts.

Serotonin neurones which assist to form the raphe nuclei, also dissipate fibres upwardly from the raphe dorsalis to the thalamus. Hence, serotonin is operative in the brain (and pervades the ventricles) and the spinal cord via descending fibres or diffusion through the cerebrospinal fluid.

One method of testing the significance of serotonin in acupuncture analgesia or other physiological functions is by accelerating its synthesis and observing any pursuant effects. In Chinese experiments reported by Han and colleagues,[26,33] the serotonin precurser 5-hydroxytryptophan (5HTP) was injected intraventricularly and intrathecally in rats with both cases resulting in an increase in the analgesic effect of acupuncture.[34] It is also possible to block the reabsorption of serotonin at the serotonergic nerve terminals. This results in an increase in availability of serotonin for receptor sites and consequently accentuates serotonergic functional activities. In a double blind study reported by Han JS and colleagues,[26] clomipramine was used to selectively block the reabsorption of serotonin and was found to be effective in increasing the level of acupuncture analgesia.[35]

Conversely, in experiments on rabbits and rats, preventing the synthesis of serotonin by injecting parachlorophenylalanine (PCPA) resulted in the attenuation of acupuncture analgesia.[34,36] Significantly though, acupuncture analgesia was not abolished totally by the injection of PCPA, implying that serotonin is not the sole determinant of the analgesic response despite its major importance.

The analgesic effect of acupuncture can be enhanced or lowered by the corresponding increase or decrease of serotonin level in the central nervous system. The implication of the results of these experiments is that serotonin in the central nervous system may be one of the most important neurochemical agents mediating acupuncture analgesia. Serotonin, which is capable of acting as a hormone and neurotransmitter, is found outside the central nervous system in a number of tissues including blood platelets and intestinal mucosa. It is interesting to note that electroacupuncture performed on patients with chronic pain also raises the platelet serotonin level significantly.[37] Just how widespread a physiological role serotonin plays (aside from analgesia) is still being explored.

It is known that patients with depression have low central and platelet serotonin levels.[38,39,40(p146)] Furthermore, these low serotonin levels are associated with greater risk of suicide.[41] Serotonin deficiencies have also been proposed as a factor in obesity. A multitude of other physiological properties are ascribed to it including the inhibition of gastric secretion, stimulation of smooth muscle, and the production of vasoconstriction.[42]

Changes of serotonin levels under acupuncture are clearly capable of exerting profound physiological responses. The influence of acupuncture on central serotonin levels may offer some explanation in western medical terms for acupuncture's beneficial effect in conditions typified by poor blood supply to the extremities such as in Raynaud's disease and diabetic polyneuropathy.[43]

Severe insomnia where both rapid eye movement (REM) and non-REM sleep are affected also follows as a consequence of depletion of serotonin in neurones in the raphe nuclei. This insomnia can be alleviated with the administration of 5-hydroxytryptophan, the precurser of serotonin.[44] In a similar fashion neurones of the locus coeruleus, another cell group in the brainstem, contain large amounts of noradrenalin. If this cell group is destroyed REM sleep is eliminated.

Locus coeruleus

We shall now turn our attention to experiments that explore the significance of noradrenalin in acupuncture. The nucleus locus coeruleus consists to a significant degree of neurones using noradrenalin(NA) (norepinephrine) as its chemical transmitter and from here fibres are sent to the forebrain and the spinal cord (ascending and descending noradrenergic fibres—see Fig. 5.4). As part of the ascending pathway, noradrenergic terminals in the raphe magnus, nucleus habenula and the PAG come mainly from the locus coeruleus. It was observed by Cao Xiaoding, Xu Shaofeng and Lu Wenxiao that electroacupuncture on human subjects and conscious rabbits decreases available noradrenalin in the brain and in the plasma suggesting that electroacupuncture inhibits the central noradrenergic system.[45] As reduced noradrenalin activity accompanied a rise in the pain threshold, Cao Xiaoding and colleagues proposed that the inhibition of sympathetic activities by acupuncture plays a favourable role in acupuncture analgesia. The inhibition of the sympathetic nervous system under electroacupuncture was also confirmed by accompanying changes in physiological indices such as palm skin temperature. Similar results have been determined for dopamine, another principal catecholomine transmitter of the sympathetic nervous system.[46,47]

The Research Group of Acupuncture Anaesthesia (Beijing) observed that increases in the cerebral content of noradrenalin were correlated with a decline in acupuncture anaesthesia and vice versa.[46] By injecting rats intraventricularly with dihydroxyphenylserine (DOPS), a presursor to NA, it was apparent that the increase in brain noradrenalin was antagonistic to the acupuncture analgesic effect. In other experiments Dun, Jiang and Fu augmented the acupuncture analgesic effect by causing chemical lesion of the noradrenergic terminals in the nucleus raphe by 6-OH-Dopamine.[48]

Cao Xiaoding and colleagues also measured a paradoxical increase due to acupuncture in noradrenalin content in the dorsal horn of the spinal cord.[45,50] Here is appears that noradrenalin plays a contradictory role. These and similar tests indicate noradrenalin in the spinal cord is an important facilitator of the acupuncture effect, that is, it augments the analgesic response.

By employing agonists and antagonists to specific receptors the Beijing research group demonstrated that central noradrenalin exerts its antagonistic effect on acupuncture analgesia specifically via alpha (adrenergic) receptors, whilst it exerts an augmentary effect via the beta-receptors. This was confirmed by others where microinjection of clonidine-M, an alpha agonist, into the periaqueductal grey could reduce the acupuncture analgesic effect.[49] (Clonidine-M encourages the functional activity of noradrenalin by increasing the susceptibility of alpha (adrenergic) receptors). The overall outcome of these experiments on rats and rabbits indicates that in the context of the function of noradrenalin, the alpha-receptor effect predominates to hinder acupuncture analgesia.

Therefore experimental evidence indicates that noradrenalin has a different role to play in different parts of the nervous system, and relates differentially to specific receptors. The balance between its actions in the brain and the spinal cord is that noradrenalin suppresses acupuncture analgesia. Of course this may vary from one species to the next, depending in part on the proliferation of alpha or beta receptors.

Studies reveal that electroacupuncture stimulation accelerates synthesis of central noradrenalin as well as its release for utilisation. But the rate of release

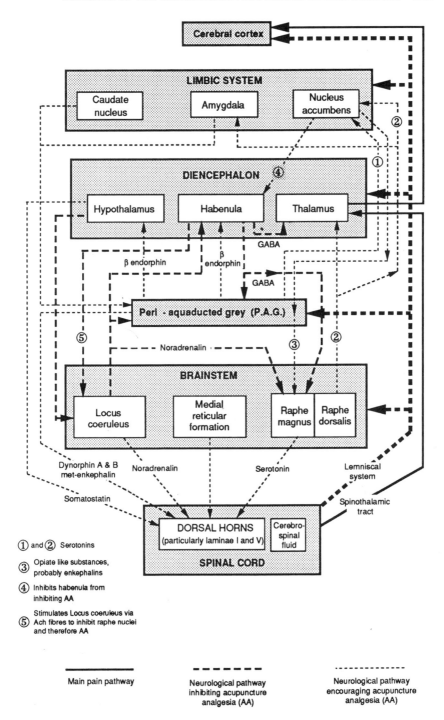

Fig. 5.4 Some of the neurological connections between the brainstem and the diencephalon that are activated by acupuncture.

exceeds that of synthesis, resulting eventually in a decrease in cerebral noradrenalin content, and therefore a weaker antagonistic effect on acupuncture analgesia, than may be anticipated. This is especially so when we consider the combined contrasting facilitatory effects of serotonin and the opiate like substances.

Periaqueductal central gray (PAG)

In order to understand properly the interrelationships between the catecholamines and opiates we need to turn our attention now to the central nervous regions in which the endogenous opiates play a significant role. The periaqueductal central grey region lies rostral to the raphe nuclei and is very important in morphine analgesia, hence has been a common and lucrative focus for research into acupuncture analgesia. As mentioned earlier, studies have identified the coexistence of serotonin and noradrenalin in the PAG, supplementary to its opioid peptidergic system.[50] The PAG, along with the nucleus accumbens, amygdaloid nucleus, and habenula (all higher in the central nervous system), and even the dorsal horns of the spinal cord have been shown by studies to represent central nervous regions with a significant presence of opioid receptors, and hence to have an important role to play in morphine or acupuncture analgesia.[18,32,51,52]

Using rats and the tailflick latency test as an estimate of pain threshold. Takeshige and fellow workers[53] confirmed earlier work by both Mayer[54] and Pomeranz[55] that acupuncture analgesia is antagonised in a dose dependent fashion by naloxone. They also concluded that acupuncture analgesia is largely mediated by opiate like substances released by activation of the dorsal PAG. Furthermore, morphine injection or electrical stimulation of the PAG can inhibit the nociceptive response of the dorsal horn neurones in the spinal cord via the descending serotonergic pathways.[17,56,57,58,59]

Radiommunoassays, which measure the amount of endogenous opioids, are also often used to establish the importance and location of opioid peptides. This information is then related to the acupuncture analgesic effect.[50,51,60] By employing opiate antagonists, synthesisers or degradation inhibitors, or radioimmunoassay techniques, different opioid peptides have been found to be present in the PAG including beta-endorphins, enkephalin, and dynorphin, each acting on different opioid receptors. The anti-nociceptive properties of beta-endorphin when injected intraventricularly are considerably more potent than morphine.[61,62] In fact, Han Jisheng claims that the anti-nociceptive nature of beta-endorphin is about 20 times more potent that that of morphine.[7] This is in contrast to the properties of enkephalins which are relatively weak anodynes despite their high affinity for opiate receptors.[63,64] It has been proposed that this weak anodyne property of the enkephalins may due to their rapid inactivation by the peptidases. Considerably less is known about the physiological characteristics of dynorphin.[21,65,66] Studies in China[7] have shown that:

weak

1. Enkephalins work in the brain, particularly the PAG and hypothalamus,[60] and the spinal cord;

powerful

2. Beta-endorphins work in the brain, but insignificantly in the spinal cord. They are particularly concentrated in the arcuate nucleus of the hypothalamus, although also present in the PAG and diencephalon;

3. Dynorphin works in the spinal cord and not in the brain; and

well known

4. Dynorphin A, followed by dynorphin B, and then met-enkephalin have a decreasing effect as opioid peptides in the spinal cord.

Cerebral opiate activity is closely correlated with acupuncture analgesia.[26] However, opiate like substances are released by the pituitary and can also at times traverse the blood-brain barrier. Blood opiate activity has also been found to be well correlated with acupuncture analgesia.[67] Cross-circulation experiments on pairs of rabbits have employed naloxone to identify the active transfer of opiates, specifically endorphins, as responsible for communication of the analgesic response.[68]

Endorphins, with their ubiquitous existence throughout the central nervous system, have provided to date a very popular theory for the mechanism of acupuncture, but as we can see from the whole range of associated neurohormones already discussed, it cannot be the complete answer. Without necessarily negating the significance of endorphins, criticisms proposed are that certain physiological responses would be expected if opiate substances played such a significant role in analgesia. Specifically, morphine and opiate like substances cause constriction of pupils (miosis), and respiratory depression, neither of which are observed in acupuncture analgesia, despite raised opiate levels. Note that the levels of opiate like substances are raised to a degree of analgesia comparible to doses of morphine that would cause these responses. Furthermore, acupuncture helps constipation, bronchospasm and gastrointestinal spasm, whilst the opiate substances do the opposite.

In response to these problems, Pasternak presents evidence suggesting that acupuncture analgesia due to endogenous opiates is mediated through a single subclass of receptor sites distinct from those mediating respiratory effects and associated with morphine mortality.[69] The opiate receptor mu-1 sites which are favoured by endogenous opioids and enkephalins appear to mediate analgesia whilst separate classes of opiate receptor sites are involved with other opiate actions. Of course, the simultaneous stimulation of other neurotransmitters may also act to diminish these expected opiate responses.

INTERACTION AT THE LEVEL OF THE DIENCEPHALON

The diencephalon, representing the posterior part of the forebrain, contains three neuronal structures that are engaged in the process of acupuncture analgesia. They are the thalamus, the habenula and the arcuate nucleus of the hypothalamus.

The thalamus

After passage through the dorsal horns of the spinal cord, the thalamic synapses are the second principal link in the afferent pain pathway. As such, the thalamus is an important site where acupuncture may exert an influence to modify noxious stimuli. And it is flush with opiate receptors.[70]

Experiments on rabbits, rats and cats showed that pain responses of neurones in the nucleus parafascicularis and nucleus centralis lateralis of the thalamus could be inhibited by acupuncture stimulation.[9,71,72,73,74] At least three quarters of the neurones measured in these two nuclei in adult cats exhibited a decrease in nociceptive discharge with electroacupuncture.[72] In the nucleus anterior and the nucleus lateralis anterior in the thalamus of rabbits similar attenuation of nociceptive responses was found to be partly mediated by endogenous opioid peptides and opioid receptors.[73]

The ascending serotonergic fibres from the raphe dorsalis are also likely to have significant input to pain modulation by acupuncture at the level of the thalamus however little research appears to be available on this topic.

Glutamic acid, an excitatory neurotransmitter, has been found in the thalamus, limbic system (hippocampus) and cerebral cortex and there is some evidence to say that it may also play a role in acupuncture analgesia.[75,76,77] Furthermore, GABA (gamma aminobutyric acid) also has an important and similarly excitatory role to play in acupuncture analgesia, and is readily converted to glutamic acid.[75] However, the habenula appears to be the most significant domain where GABA exerts its influence.

Habenula

The habenula, in the dorsomedial aspect of the thalamus, is a relay station between the limbic system and the lower brainstem.

I have already briefly made mention of the habenula as a site where opioids are found in an aspect supportive of acupuncture analgesia.[78] However, other studies have shown that during electroacupuncture analgesia the habenula inhibits the analgesic responses in the PAG,[79] the thalamus,[77] and the raphe nuclei[76] by releasing GABA (gamma amino-butyric acid) (Figure 5.4). GABA in the brain is antagonistic to acupuncture analgesia, that is, an increase in GABA (which excites neuronal activity) results in a decrease in analgesia.

Not only does the habenula inhibit the (acupuncture) analgesic effect of the PAG and raphe nuclei via GABA fibres, but it also acts to stimulate the locus coeruleus (via cholinergic fibres) to inhibit the raphe nuclei further.[7] Inhibition of the raphe nuclei by the locus coeruleus is achieved through the noradrenergic pathways already discussed. Hence, acupuncture is capable of increasing the release of GABA particularly in the habenula where in turn it is able to exert inhibitory actions on acupuncture analgesia directly via the raphe nuclei, and indirectly via cholinergic fibres to the locus coeruleus. In disease states the impairment of GABA transmission may modify the acetylcholine and monoamine systems to promote sleep disorders and may produce a variety of seizure disorders, including grand mal fits.[40]

Arcuate nucleus of the hypothalamus

The arcuate nucleus of the hypothalamus is also a site for beta-endorphin neurones, which in turn travel to the PAG and locus coeruleus in the brainstem and hence facilitate acupuncture analgesia at these levels.[80,81,82,83]

Yin Qizhang and colleagues at the Suzhou Medical College illustrated in elaborate controlled experiments on rats that electroacupuncture could activate the arcuate neurones with the result of inhibiting their noxious responses.[80] Painful stimuli could elicit evoked potentials in the arcuate nucleus, which were subsequently inhibited by electroacupuncture. Separate tests also showed that electrical stimulation of the arcuate nucleus could enhance the analgesic effect of acupuncture whilst lesion or isolation of this nucleus would reduce the acupuncture analgesic effect.

Aside from beta-endorphin neurones, experiments have confirmed that cholinergic neurones also have a role to play in the analgesic and regulatory effect of acupuncture in the hypothalamus.[84,85] Increased hypothalamic acetylcholine (Ach) levels are positively correlated with the analgesic outcome.

Experiments on rats in Beijing used the tailflick test as an estimate of pain threshold to determine that acupuncture analgesia could be attenuated by inhibiting the synthesis of acetylcholine with intraventricular hemicholine injections or by introducing the receptor antagonist, atropine. The effect of hemicholine could be partially reversed by the administration of the acetycholine precurser, choline. On the other hand injections of eserine, an anticholinesterase which assists the central accumulation of acetylcholine, potentiated acupuncture analgesia.[86,87] Many regions other than the arcuate nucleus of the hypothalamus, have been found that involve acetycholine in the acupuncture analgesia pathway, such as the caudate nucleus,[47] the amygdala, the habenula, the cortex and particularly the locus coeruleus.[85,86,88]

THE LIMBIC SYSTEM

The main structures to be discussed here for their part in the acupuncture ensemble are the nucleus accumbens, amygdala, and caudate nucleus.

Nucleus accumbens

The nucleus accumbens is an important neuronal structure which is supplied by serotonin fibres from the PAG and the raphe dorsalis (Fig. 5.4 pathways 1 and 2).[7] Release of serotonin in the nucleus accumbens in turn activates the liberation of met-enkephalins there, which act to promote analgesia. From the nucleus accumbens a descending pathway to the nucleus raphe utilises these endogenous opioids as neurotransmitters (Fig. 5.4 pathway 3). This descending pathway which terminates in the nucleus raphe, acts to further inhibit pain signals there and supports analgesia. Any inhibition at the level of the raphe nuclei of the ascending serotonergic channels to the nucleus accumbens would decrease the level of acupuncture induced analgesia.

In Figure 5.4 these pathways just described are labelled with the numbers 1, 2, and 3, and form what is termed (tentatively by Han Jisheng) the 'meso-limbic loop of analgesia'.[7] This neuronal loop, existing between the PAG, the raphe dorsalis and nucleus accumbens, utilises serotonin and the enkephalins as neurotransmitters, and acts as a positive feedback cycle in analgesia. This feedback loop may be one reason why acupuncture analgesia lasts for some time after the removal of needles. Another factor already mentioned would be a reflection of the clearance rate (half life) of the relevant neurotransmitters from the cerebrospinal fluid and blood.

Another link which acts as a collateral to the group is labelled '4' on Figure 5.4. In this collateral of the feedback loop the nucleus accumbens sends descending impulses that inhibit the function of the habenula.[78] Descending fibres from the habenula which release GABA in the PAG and raphe nuclei would normally inhibit acupuncture analgesia, however as the habenula itself is a victim of descending inhibition from the nucleus accumbens, the influence of GABA to decrease the pain threshold would be curbed.[89]

Amygdala

Not only are opiate like substances involved in the amygdala, but serotonin fibres also pervade this area and are derived from the raphe dorsalis. In Beijing Medical College the presence of serotonin in the amygdala and its relationship to acupuncture analgesia has been tested in controlled studies on rabbits using cinanserin, a serotonin receptor blocker.[90] The opiate substances were tested with naloxone and D-phenylalnine, an enkephalin degradation enzyme inhibitor. As would be expected both serotonin and enkephalins were found to facilitate electroacupuncture analgesia. Nanjing University, by studying unit discharges of the amygdala, also confirmed the involvement of this nucleus in the modulation of pain and acupuncture.[91] They proposed that the raphe nuclei acted as a relay station for the acupuncture impulses prior to reaching the amygdala. In interesting contrast however, Zhang Anzhong in earlier studies had noted in rabbits that 'no prominent changes of endorphin release in the amygdala during acupuncture analgesia were observed' (p135).[92]

Caudate nucleus

Placed rostrally to the thalamus, the caudate nucleus also appears to participate in acupuncture analgesic effects. Experimenters in Shanghai observed that electrical stimulation of the head of the caudate nucleus provided relief from intractable pain caused by advanced tumours in all 17 patients tested.[93] Furthermore, the characteristics of analgesia induced by the electrical stimulation of the caudate nucleus closely mimicked the characteristics of acupuncture analgesia.

Other experiments performed in Shanghai First Medical College have shown that acetylcholine plays an important facilitating role in the acupuncture effect. When injected into the caudate nucleus, the cholinergic blocker, scopolamine, blocked acupuncture analgesia.[47,94,95] Furthermore, in their experiments with rabbits at the Shanghai First Medical College and elsewhere, researchers have clarified that not only acetylcholine, but dopamine, serotonin and the opiates all operate in the caudate region (Fig. 5.5).[96,97,98,99]

In fact the caudate cholinergic activity is antagonised by the release of dopamine under electroacupuncture. Though an increase in concentration of dopamine in the caudate nucleus appears to have an effect against electroacupuncture analgesia, Sun Deyu and colleagues in Jinzhou Medical College demonstrated that injection of dopamine into the substantia nigra at the level of the midbrain increased the analgesic effect induced by electroacupuncture at Zusanli (St 36).[100] Unlike its function in the caudate nucleus, dopamine in the substantia nigra operates to increase the pain threshold. Here, dopamine is the most important inhibitory neurotransmitter.[101] The behaviour of dopamine is another reminder of the contradictory roles these neurochemicals may be playing under acupuncture stimulus. The overall effect of the dopamine system is, according to Xu Shaofen, antagonistic to acupuncture analgesia.[98,99]

Having determined that acetylcholine activity in the caudate nucleus enhances acupuncture analgesia and that this may be antagonised by dopamine, Xu Zhenbang explored further for drugs that might potentiate acupuncture analgesia.[47] Metoclopramide seemed to suit the requirements as it has both anticholinesterase and antidopamine functions.[102,103] Intravenous administration of metoclopramide to rabbits enhanced the elevation and prolongation of pain threshold with electroacupuncture. This is an interesting example of how pharmaceutical drugs may be adapted to enhance the acupuncture response.

Cerebral cortex

The cerebral cortex is involved in the integration and descending modulation of pain.[104,105,106,107] It is fairly well established through morphological and other studies that the cerebral cortex employs efferent connections to a number of nuclei lower in the brain, (such as the PAG, caudate nucleus, reticular formation of midbrain, spinal cord, raphe magnus and thalamus), in order to modulate not only pain, but various other sensations.[108,109,110,111,112,113,114] The complicated modulatory effect on the subcortical structures is evidenced, for example, by the way the somatosensory area II is inhibitory to the parafasciculus nucleus in the thalamus, whereas the motor cortex is facilitatory to the same nucleus (Fig. 5.5).[7]

Corticofugal (moving away from cortex) impulses from somatosensory area II in the cortex to the centromedian nucleus (CM) in the thalamus are involved in the production and maintenance of the acupuncture analgesia

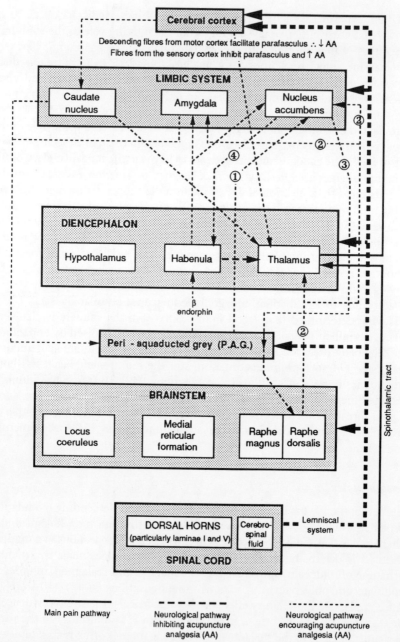

Fig. 5.5 Neurological connections activated or enhanced by acupuncture between the limbic system, diencephalon and cerebral cortex.

effect. These impulses from somatosensory area II are thought to be initiated by the acupuncture stimulus.[115,116] GABA injections in the somatosensory area II appear to suppress the cortical descending pain inhibitory effect, whilst acupuncture analgesia may be prolonged by glutamate injection in the same area.[77]

Experiments have shown that by recording unit discharges, the responses of neurones of the cerebral cortex somatosensory area I to noxious stimuli can be inhibited by electroacupuncture. Interestingly, the unit discharges due to weak rather than strong electroacupuncture could be blocked significantly by intravenous naloxone, implying that the cerebral cortex's role in acupuncture analgesia induced by weak electroacupuncture is modulated by opiate like substances.[117] In experiments with human subjects in Beijing, cerebral evoked potentials (CEP) were graphed under the presence of noxious stimuli followed by electroacupuncture.[118] Electroacupuncture induced an inhibitory effect on the components relating to pain in the cerebral evoked potentials. This experiment provides further substantial evidence of the objective reality of the analgesic effect of acupuncture.

These limited cases exemplify the complex modulatory effect the cerebral cortex exerts under acupuncture. It was mentioned earlier that noradrenalin acts in a facilitatory way in the spinal cord whilst high levels of noradrenalin in the brain negate acupuncture analgesia. In a similar fashion, the alpha and beta noradrenergic receptors adopt different roles in the context of acupuncture analgesia. And this complex interaction of just one neurotransmitter is echoed by the full spectrum of interactions of transmitter substances that play a part in the physiological responses to acupuncture.

NEUROTRANSMITTER INTERRELATIONSHIPS

Thus far it is apparent that serotonin and the opiate like substances are of major importance in acupuncture analgesia. The functions of these two substances are also very closely related. For example, it was stated earlier that opiate stimulation in the raphe magnus initiates serotonin release in the spinal cord. Hence, it may be of interest to explore the extent of mutual interaction and support between these two neurotransmitters. Studies on rats in China have shown that:[26]

1. When both central serotonin content and opiate activity levels are high, the result is excellent acupuncture analgesia. When only one factor is high, moderate analgesia usually results. When neither factors is raised, or both are blocked, the outcome is poor analgesia.[119,120]

2. Blockage of the effect of opiate receptors with intravenous naloxone obstructs the endogenous opioids and results in an increase in the turnover rate of central serotonin.

3. A decrease in central serotonin content leads to an increase in cerebral opiate activity.

The interrelationship between serotonin and the opiate like substances is important in that it may provide some insight into, and explanation of, variations in experimental results. Experiments which control or measure only serotonin or opioid activity may not arrive at the same conclusions regarding the importance of these transmitters. For example, Kenyon, Knight and Wells concluded that endorphins did not appear to be important in the mechanism of acupuncture therapy for chronic pain.[124] Total pain relief before and after a naloxone block to the acupuncture seemed unchanged indicating that the endogenous opiates in these twenty patients played no role. However, when we keep in mind the studies of Han Jisheng and colleagues, it is apparent that other neurotransmitters may well have been engaged in lieu of the opiates to bring about an overall analgesic response.

It seems clear that the mobilisation of cerebral serotonin and opiate substances are intimately related to the effect of acupuncture analgesia and (at least in animal studies) they appear to compensate each other's functions. Brain serotonin may play a more important role in the effect of acupuncture analgesia in morphine tolerant subjects. Hence, acupuncture analgesia could still be successful and therefore offer possibility of treatment to narcotic tolerant patients.

Han Jisheng and colleagues mathematically correlated the analgesic outcome of acupuncture with both central serotonin content and opiate activity.[26] They found that this correlation could be expressed in a regression equation. Their regression equation held true for normal rats and reflects the substantial relationship between serotonin, the opiates and acupuncture analgesia. In subsequent studies this equation was shown to be consistent across different experimental conditions using the same species of animal, for example, rats . . . whether healthy or sick.[26]

Acupuncture tolerance

Acupuncture tolerance is the state that occurs when acupuncture analgesia is mantained over a prolonged period. If the acupuncture analgesia stimulus were to be maintained for a few hours or more, the result would be a curtailment of the analgesic effect. This is not explicable by the possible cerebral depletion of opiate like substances as a response to excessive and prolonged release, because it has been found that cerebral opiate levels were still considerably higher than usual in the acupuncture tolerant subjects.[121] Opiate activity is still higher than normal despite the fall in analgesia, and administration of morphine to acupuncture tolerant rats induced only a minimal analgesic effect.[122]

The production in the central nervous system of anti-opiate substances (AOS) such as cholecystokinin (CKK-8: cholecystokinin octapeptide) is a logical explanation of the appearance of acupuncture tolerance. This is certainly substantiated by experiments that demonstrate that intrathecal injection of CKK–8 supresses acupuncture analgesia almost completely, or that removal of CKK-8 (via the introduction of antibodies) postpones the development of acupuncture tolerance.[7] Although reports of such experiments mainly discuss the spinal content of cholecystokinin, this transmitter, antagonistic to acupuncture analgesia, is located more significantly in the cortex, hypothalamus, limbic system, and periaqueductal grey of the brainstem and hence may exert a similar influence there.[21] The build up of other antagonists such as noradrenalin in the brain and substance P in the spinal cord may also account for some degree of acupuncture tolerance.

REFERENCES

1. Melzack R, Wall P D 1965 Pain mechanisms; a new theory. Science 150(3699): 971–978
2. Morphological Section of the Acupuncture Anaesthesia Research Unit, Shenyang Medical College 1973 Preliminary experimental morphological and electron microscopic studies of the connection between acupuncture points on the limbs and the segments of the spinal cord. Chinese Medical Journal 3: 144–150
3. Wall P D 1978 The gate control theory of pain mechanisms; a re-examination and restatement. Brain 101: 1–18
4. Melzack R, Jeans M E 1974 Acupuncture analgesia: a psychophysiological explanation. Minnesota Medicine 57(Mar): 161– 166
5. Man P L, Chen C H 1972 Mechanism of acupunctural anesthesia: the two gate control theory. Diseases of the Nervous System 33(Nov): 730–735
6. Man P L, Chen C H 1972 Acupuncture 'anesthesia': a new theory and clinical study. Current Therapeutic Research 14(7): 390–394
7. Han J S 1984 On the mechanism of acupuncture analgesia. Acupuncture Research 3(9): 236–245
8. Melzack R 1973 How acupuncture can block pain. Impact of Science on Society (UNESCO) 23(1): 65
9. Mu J 1985 Lectures communicated on the occasion of the Fourth International Advanced Studies Acupuncture Course (WHO), Nanjing
10. Fields H L, Anderson S D 1978 Evidence that raphe-spinal neurones mediate opiate and midbrain stimulation-produced analgesias. Pain 5: 333–349
11. Lovick T A, West D C, Wolstencroft J H 1978 Responses of raphespinal and other bulbar raphe neurones to stimulation of the PAG in the cat. Neuroscience Letters 8: 45
12. Chung S H, Dickenson A 1980 Pain, enkephalin and acupuncture. Nature 283(Jan): 243–244
13. Dickenson A, Oliveras J L, Besson J M 1979 Role of the nucleus raphe magnus in opiate analgesia as studied by the microinjection technique in the rat. Brain Research 170: 95–111
14. Yaksh T L, Rudy T A 1979 Narcotic analgesics: CNS sites and mechanisms of action as revealed by intracerebral injection techniques. Pain 4: 299–359
15. Yaksh T L, Tyce G M 1979 Microinjection of morphine into the periaquaductal grey evokes the release of serotonin from spinal cord. Brain Research 171:176–181
16. Rivot J P, Chaouch A, Besson J M 1979 The influence of naloxone on the C-fibre response of dorsal horn neurons and their inhibitory control by raphe magnus stimulation. Brain Research 176: 355–364
17. Oliveras J L, Hosobuchi Y, Redjemi F, Guilbaud G, Besson J M 1977 Opiate antagonist naloxone strongly reduces analgesia induced by stimulation of a raphe nucleus (centralis inferior). Brain Research 120: 221–229
18. Hokfelt T, Elde R, Johansson O, Luft R, Nilsson C, Arimura A 1976 Immunohistochemical evidence for separate populations of somatostatin-containing and substance P-containing primary afferent neurones in the rat. Neuroscience 1:131–136
19. Hokfelt T, Johansson O, Kellerth J O, Ljungdahl A, Nilsson G, Nygards A, Pernow B 1977 Immunohistochemical distribution of SP. In: von Euler US, Pernow B (eds) Substance P. Raven Press, New York p 117–145

20. Randic M, Miletic V 1978 Depressant actions of methionine- enkephalin and somatostatin in cat dorsal horn neurones activated by noxious stimuli. Brain Research 152: 196–202
21. Abrams G M, Recht L 1982 Neuropeptides and their role in pain and analgesia. Acupuncture and Electrotherapeutics Research 7: 105–121
22. Otsuka M, Konishi S 1976 Release of substance P-like immunoreactivity from isolated spinal cord of the newborn rat. Nature 264: 83–84
23. Needham J, Lu G D 1980 Celestial lancets: a history and rationale of acupuncture and moxibustion. Cambridge University Press, Cambridge
24. Oehme P, Hilse H, Morgenstern E, Gores E 1980 Substance P: does it produce analgesia or hyperalgesia? Science 208: 305–307
25. Frederickson R C A, Burgis V, Harrell C E, Edwards J D 1978 Dual actions of substance P on nociception: possible role of endogenous opioids. Science 199: 1359–1362
26. Han J S, Tang J, Ren M F, Zhou Z F, Fan S G, Qiu X S 1980 Central neurotransmitters and acupuncture analgesia. American Journal of Chinese Medicine 8(4): 331–348
27. Behbehani M M(1) 1978 Effect of morphine injected in PAG on the activity of single units in RM of the rat. Brain Research 149: 266–269
28. Behbehani M M(2) 1979 Evidence that an excitatory connection between the PAG and nucleus raphe magnus mediates stimulation produced analgesia. Brain Research 170: 85–93
29. Pomeroy S L, Behbehani M M 1979 Physiologic evidence for a projection from periaqueductal grey to nucleus raphe magnus in the rat. Brain Research 176: 143–147
30. Zhu L X, Shi Q Y 1984 Activation of nucleus raphe magnus by acupuncture and enkephinergic nechanism. Journal of Traditional Chinese Medicine 4(2): 111–113
31. Simantov R, Kuhar M J, Pasternak G W, Snyder S H 1976 The regional distribution of a morphinelike factor enkephalin in monkey brain. Brain Research 106: 189–197
32. Kuhar M, Pert C, Snyder S 1973 Regional distribution of opiate receptor binding in monkey and human brain. Nature 245: 447–450
33. Han J S, Chou P H, Lu L H, Yang T H, Jen M F 1979 The role of central 5–hydroxytryptamine in acupuncture analgesia. Scientia Sinica 22: 91–104
34. Anon(1) 1976 Effect of p-chlorophenylalanine and 5– hydroxytryptophan on acupuncture analgesia in rats. Journal of New Medical Pharmacology 3: 133–138 (in Chinese). Reported in Han J S, Tang J, Ren M F, Zhou Z F, Fan S G, Qiu X C (see Biblio No 26 above)
35. Zhao F Y, Meng X Z, Yu S D, Ma A H, Dong X Y, Han C S 1978 Impacted last molar extraction under finger pressing anesthesia: effect of clomipramine and pargyline. Journal of the Peking Medical College 2: 79–82 (in Chinese). In: Han J S, Tang J, Ren M F, Zhou Z F, Fan S G, Qiu X S (see Biblio No reference 26 above)
36. Anon(2) 1974 Effect of p-chlorophenylalanine on acupuncture analgesia in rabbits. Kexue Tongbao 20: 483–485 (in Chinese). Reported in Han J S, Tang J, Ren M F, Zhou Z F, Fan S G, Qiu X C (reference 26)
37. Mao W, Ghia J N, Scott D S, Duncan G H, Gregg J M 1980 High versus low intensity acupuncture analgesia for treatment of chronic pain: effects on platelet serotonin. Pain 8: 331–342
38. Sternbach R A, Janowsky D S, Huey L Y, Segal D S 1976 Effects altering brain serotonin in activity on human chronic pain. In: Bonica J J, Albe-Fessard D (eds), Advances in Pain Research and Therapy 1: 601–606. Raven Press, New York
39. Sarai K, Kayano M 1968 The level and diurnal rhythm of serum serotonin in manic-depressive patients. Folia Psychiatrica et Neurologica Japonica 22: 271–278
40. Patterson M 1986 Hooked? NET: the new approach to drug cure. Faber & Faber, London
41. van Praag H M 1983 Depression. Lancet 2: 912
42. Miller B F, Keane C B 1983 Encyclopeadia and dictionary of medicine, nursing and allied health, 3rd edn. Saunders, Philadelphia
43. Kaada B, Eielsen O 1983 In search of mediators of skin vasodilation induced by transcutaneous nerve stimulation: II Serotonin implicated. General Pharmacology 14: 635–641
44. Schmidt R F(ed) 1978 Fundamentals of neurophysiology. Springer Verlag, New York
45. Cao X D, Xu S F, Lu W X 1983 Inhibition of symathetic nervous system by acupuncture. Acupuncture and Electrotherapeutics Research 8: 25–35
46. Research group of Acupuncture Anaesthesia, Peking Medical College 1979 The role of central catecholamines in acupuncture anaesthesia. Chinese Medical Journal 92: 793–800
47. Xu Z B, Pan Y Y, Xu S F, Mo W Y, Cao X D, He L F 1983 Synergism between metoclopramide and EAA. Acupuncture and Electrotherapeutics Research 8: 283–288

48. Dun S W, Jiang J F, Fu L W 1979 Influences of intracerebral injection
    of 6–OH-Dopamine on acupuncture analgesia and monoamine neurons' histoflurescence
    of dorsal raphe nucleus. Acta Physiologia Sinica 31: 273–280.
49. Zhou Z F, Du M Y, Wu W Y, Han J S 1979 The effect of the injection of naloxone into
    habenula or amygdala on AA in the rabbit. National Symposium on Acupuncture,
    Moxibustion and Acupuncture Anaesthesia, Beijing Paper No 504
50. Cao X D, He L F, Xu X F et al 1984 The role of PAG in AA. Second National Symposium
    of Acupuncture and Moxibustion and Acupuncture Anaesthesia, Beijing Paper No 639
51. Simantov R, Childers S R, Snyder S H 1977 Opioid peptides: differentiation by
    radioimmunoassay and radioreceptor assay. Brain Research 135: 358–367
52. He L F, Dong W Q 1983 Activity of opioid peptidergic system in acupuncture analgesia.
    Acupuncture and Electrotherapeutics Research 8: 257–266
53. Takeshige C, Sato T, Komugi H 1980 Role of PA central G in AA. Acupuncture and
    Electrotherapeutics Research 5: 323–337
54. Mayer D J, Price D D, Raffii A 1977 Antagonism of acupuncture analgesia in man by the
    narcotic antagonist naloxone. Brain Research 121:368–372
55. Pomeranz B, Chiu 1976 Naloxone blockade of acupuncture analgesia: endorphin
    implicated. Life Sciences 19: 1757–1762
56. Reynolds D V 1969 Surgery in the rat during electrical analgesia induced by focal brain
    stimulation. Science 164: 444
57. Mayer D J, Wolfe T L, Akil H, Carder B, Liebeskind J C 1971 Analgesia from electrical
    stimulation in the brainstem of the rat. Science 174: 1351–1354
58. Carstens E, Yokota T, Zimmerman M 1979 Inhibition of spinal neuronal responses to
    noxious skin heating by stimulation of mesencephalic periaqueductal grey in the cat.
    Journal of Neurophysiology 42(2): 558
59. Bennet G J, Mayer D J 1979 Inhibition of spinal cord interneurones by narcotic
    microinjection and focal electrical stimulation in the periaqueductal central grey matter.
    Brain Research 172: 243–257
60. Shanghai Institute of Materia Medica 1979 Radioimmunoassay for enkephalins. National
    Symposium on Acupuncture, Moxibustion and Acupuncture Anaesthesia, Beijing Paper
    Nos 488–490
61. Loh H H, Tseng L F, Wei E, Li C H 1976 B-endorphin is a potent analgesic agent.
    Proceedings of the National Academy of Science (USA) 73: 2895–2898
62. Feldberg W, Smyth D G 1976 The C-fragment of lipotropin - a potent analgesic. Journal of
    Physiology 260: 30P-31P
63. Beluzzi J D, Grant N, Garsley V, Sarantakis D, Wise C D, Stein L 1976 Analgesia induced
    in vivo by central administration of enkephalin in rat. Nature 260: 625–626
64. Chang J K, Fong T W 1976 Opiate receptor affinities and behavioural effects of
    enkephalin: structure activity relationship of ten synthetic peptide analogues. Life
    Sciences 18: 1473–1481
65. Goldstein A S, Tachabana S, Lowney L I, Hunkapiller M, Hood L 1979 Dynorphin
    (1–13), an extraordinary potent opioid peptide. Proceedings of the National Academy
    Science (USA) 76: 6666–6669
66. Friedman H J, Jen M F, Chang J K, Lee N M, Loh H H 1981 Dynorphin: a possible
    modulatory peptide on morphine or B-endorphin analgesia in mouse. European Journal of
    Pharmacology 69: 357–360
67. Xu S L, Fu Z L, Ziang M J et al 1979 The effect of AA and its relation to blood endorphin,
    blood histamine, and suggestibility. National Symposium on Acupuncture, Moxibustion
    and Acupuncture Anaesthesia, Beijing Paper No 510
68. Yang M M P, Kok S H 1979 Further study of the neurohumoral factor, endorphin, in the
    mechanism of AA. American Journal of Chinese Medicine 7(2): 143–148
69. Pasternak G W 1981 Central mechanisms of opioid analgesia. Acupuncture and
    Electrotherapeutics Research 6: 135–149
70. Chang K J, Cooper B R, Hazum E, Cuatrecasas P 1979 Multiple opiate receptors:
    Differential regional distribution in the brain and differential binding of opiates and opioid
    peptides. Molecular Pharmacology 16: 91–104
71. Chang H T 1973 Integrative action of thalamus in the process of acupuncture for analgesia.
    Scientica Sinica 16(1): 25–60
72. Xu W, Lin Y, Chen Z Q, Zhang Y F 1984 The effect of EA points on nociceptive
    responses of Pf and CM neurones of the thalamus. Second National Symposium on
    Acupuncture, Moxibustion and Acupuncture Anaesthesia, Beijing Paper No 350

73. He L F, Wang M Z 1984 Effect of EA on evoked response of neurones in N. Anterior and N. Lateralis anterior of thalamus of rabbit. Second National Symposium of Acupuncture and Moxibustion and Acupuncture Anaesthesia, Beijing Paper No 380
74. Zhao Z Q, Shao D H, Yang Z Q 1986 Inhibition of evoked discharges of posterior nuclear group of thalamus induced by stimulation of central grey matter, caudate nucleus and electroacupuncture in waking rabbits. In: Zhang X T (ed) Research on acupuncture, moxibustion, and acupuncture anesthesia. Science Press, Beijing
75. Zhu J Q, Li C B, Xu F, Liang W J 1984 Relationship of the metabolism of GABA in mice brain to electroacupuncture analgesia. Second National Symposium on Acupuncture, Moxibustion and Acupuncture Anaesthesia, Beijing Paper No 490
76. Wang S, Liu G, Liu W, Gao Y, Tang Y 1987 Habenula and acupuncture analgesia. World Federation of Acupuncture and Moxibustion Societies, First World Conference, 1987 Compilation of Abstracts of Papers, p215-217
77. Second National Symposium on Acupuncture, Moxibustion and Acupuncture Anaesthesia, 1984, Beijing Paper Nos 352,353
78. Fan S G, Tang J, Ren M F et al 1979 The effect of injection of naloxone into nucleus accumbens and habenula on AA in the rat. National Symposium of Acupuncture and Moxibustion and Acupuncture Anaesthesia, Beijing Paper No 505
79. Fang J Z, Wang S, Xia Y H 1984 The influence of habenula on periaqueductal grey matter in AA. Second National Symposium of Acupuncture and Moxibustion and Acupuncture Anaesthesia, Beijing Paper No 398
80. Yin Q Z, Duanma Z X, Guo S Y, Yu X M, Zhang Y J 1984 Role of the hypothalamic arcuate nucleus in AA; A review of behavioural and electrophysiological studies. Journal of Traditional Chinese Medicine 4(2): 103-110
81. Finley J C W, Lindstrom P, Petrusz P 1981 Immunocytochemical localisation of beta-endorphin-containing neurones in the rat brain. Neuroendocrinology 33(1): 28-42
82. Gao Y S, Gu Y H 1984 Mechanism underlying the inhibitory effect of nucleus arcuatus hypothalami on unit discharge of locus coeruleus with reference to EA. Second National Symposium of Acupuncture and Moxibustion and Acupuncture Anaesthesia, Beijing Paper No 391
83. Gao Y S, Gu Y H 1984 Mechanism underlying the excitatory effect of nucleus arcuatus hypothalami on PAG-NRM system and its significance in EA. Second National Symposium of Acupuncture and Moxibustion and Acupuncture Anaesthesia, Beijing Paper No 392
84. Tang J X, Lu C H, Huang X Y, Sun H Q 1979 The influence of electroacupuncture anaesthesia on cholinergic transmitter in patients and rats. National Symposium on Acupuncture, Moxibustion and Acupuncture Anaesthesia, Beijing Paper No 451
85. Wang C Y, Yu B, Liu X C 1979 The influence of acupuncture on the Ach level in variuos regions of rat brain. National Symposium on Acupuncture, Moxibustion and Acupuncture Anaesthesia, Beijing Paper No 453
86. Ren M F, Tu Z P, Han J S 1979 The effect of hemicholine, choline, eserine and atropine on AA in the rat. National Symposium of Acupuncture, Moxibustion and Acupuncture Anaesthesia, Beijing Paper No 450
87. Guan X M, Yu B, Wang C Y, Liu X C 1986 Role of cholinergic nerves in electroacupuncture analgesia—influence of acetylcholine, eserine, neostigmine, and hemicholinum on electroacupuncture analgesia. In: Zhang X T (ed) 1986 Research on acupuncture, moxibustion, and acupuncture anaesthesia. Science Press, Beijing
88. Ai M K, Wu Z J, Li T P 1986 Influence of electroacupuncture on ultrastructure of synapses in medial region of rat thalamus. In: Zhang X T (ed) 1986 Research on Acupuncture, Moxibustion, and acupuncture anaesthesia. Science Press, Beijing
89. Wang S, Fang J, Xia Y 1984 The role of nucleus accumbens stimulation on discharges of the PAG matter in AA. National Symposium on Acupuncture, Moxibustion and Acupuncture Anaesthesia, Beijing Paper No 397
90. Xu D, Zhou Z, Xie G, Han J 1984 Amygdala: its importance in mediating EAA and morphine analgesia. Second National Symposium on Acupuncture, Moxibustion and Acupuncture Anaesthesia, Beijing Paper No 376
91. Sun G, Wang J, Yin S 1984 The influence of EA and electrical stimulation of midbrain raphe on unit activity of amygdala in awake, unrested rabbits. Second National Symposium on Acupuncture, Moxibustion and Acupuncture Anaesthesia, Beijing Paper No 377

92. Zhang A Z 1980 Endorphin and acupuncture analgesia research in the People's Republic of China (1975-1979). Acupuncture and Electrotherapeutics Research 5: 131-146
93. Chen G B, Jiang C C, Li S C et al 1982 The role of the human caudate nucleus in AA. Acupuncture and Electrotherapeutics Research 7: 255-265
94. He L F, Xu S F 1981 Caudate nucleus and acupuncture analgesia. Acupuncture and Electrotherapeutics Research 6:169-182
95. He L, Ho X, Si C 1979 Effect of intracaudate microinjection of scopolamine on EA in the rabbit. Acta Physiologia Sinica 31: 47-52
96. Ladinsky H, Consolo S, Bianchi S, Samanin R, Ghezzi D 1975 Cholinergic-dopaminergic interaction in the striatum: the effect of 6-Hydroxydopamine or pimozide treatment on the increased striatal acetylcholine levels induced by apomorphine, piribedil and d-amphetamine. Brain Research 84: 221-226
97. Portig P J, Vogt M 1969 Release into the cerebral ventricles of substances with a possible transmitter function in the caudate nucleus. Journal of Physiology 204: 687-715
98. Xu S F, Lu W X, Zhou G Z, Sheng M P, Wang D L 1984 Effects of cholinergic and dopaminergic systems of the caudate nucleus in AA. Second National Symposium on Acupuncture, Moxibustion and Acupuncture Anaesthesia, Beijing Paper No 471
99. Xu S F 1978 The influence of acupuncture on the acetylcholine level in the brain. Scientia Sinica 23: 572
100. Sun D Y, Wang W Q, Jiang E K, Gao D M 1984 Effect of intrasubstantia nigra injection of dopamine on EAA in rabbits. Second National Symposium on Acupuncture, Moxibustion and Acupuncture Anaesthesia, Beijing Paper No 479
101. Gilman S, Winams S 1983 Essentials of clinical neuroanatomy and neurophysiology, 6th edn. FA Davis, Philadelphia
102. Karanth K S, Gurumadhra Rao S, Padma Kumari T K, Guruswami M N 1981 Anticholinesterase activity of metoclopramide. Indian Journal of Medical Research 74:125-128
103. Schulze-Delrien K 1981 Metoclopramide. New England Journal of Medicine 305: 28-33
104. DelgadoJ M R 1955 Cerebral structures involved in transmission and elaboration of noxious stimulation. Journal of Neurophysiology 18: 261
105. Berkley K J, Palmer R 1974 Somatosensory cortical involvement in responses to noxious stimulation in the cat. Experimental Brain Research 20: 363-374
106. Xu W, Chen Z, Lin Y 1986 On the involvment of the cerebral cortex in descending modulation of pain and analgesia. Journal of Traditional Chinese Medicine 6(4): 279-288
107. Chen Z, Xu W, Lin Y 1986 Identification of cortico-thalamic neurons: involvement of corticol descending modulation in acupuncture analgesia. Journal of Traditional Chinese Medicine 6(3): 195-200
108. Soto-Moyano R, Hernandez A 1981 Morphine induced cortical excitation and its influence on thalamic somatosensory evoked activity. Archives Internationales de Pharmacodynamie 254(2): 214-222
109. Kuypers H G J M, Lawrence D G 1967 Cortical projections to the red nucleus and the brain stem in the rhesus monkey. Brain Research 4: 151-188
110. Brown A G, Coulter J D, Rose P K, Short A D, Snow P J 1977 Inhibition of spinocervical tract discharges from localised areas of the sensorimotor cortex in the cat. Journal of Physiology (Lond) 264: 1-16
111. Yezierski R P, Gerhart K D, Schrock B J, Willis W D 1983 A further examination of effects of cortical stimulation on primate spinothalamic tract cells. Journal of Neurophysiology 49(2): 424
112. Oka H 1980 Organisation of cortico-caudate projections: a HRP study in the cat. Brain Research 40: 203
113. Royce G J 1983 Cell of origin of corticothalamic projections upon the centromedian and parafascicular nuclei in the cat. Brain Research 258: 11-21
114. Kunzle H 1977 Projection from the primary somatosensory cortex to basal ganglia and thalamus in the monkey. Experimental Brain Research 30: 481-492
115. Lin Y, Xu W 1984 The function of corticofugal impulses of SII on the inhibitory effect of acupuncture at CM. Second National Symposium on Acupuncture, Moxibustion and Acupuncture Anaesthesia, Beijing Paper No 354
116. Lin Y, Xu W 1984 Corticofugal impulses of SII involved in the regulation of nociceptive response of CM and its interrelation with acupuncture effect. Second National Symposium on Acupuncture, Moxibustion and Acupuncture Anaesthesia, Beijing Paper No 355

117. Dong W C, Xu W, Chen Z Q et al 1984 The influence of acupuncture on responses of neurons in the cerebral cortex to noxious stimuli and the effect of naloxone. Second National Symposium of Acupuncture and Moxibustion and Acupuncture Anaesthesia, Beijing Paper No 357
118. Xia L Y, Huang K H, Zhao W F, Rong X D, Xu W B, Liang X S 1984 The inhibitory effects of electroacupuncture on cerebral evoked potential and the model graph of cerebral pain evoked potential of human. Second National Symposium on Acupuncture, Moxibustion and Acupuncture Anaesthesia, Beijing Paper No 348
119. Han J S, Tang J, Fan S G et al 1986 Central 5-Hydroxytrptamine, opiate-like substance and acupuncture analgesia. In: Zhang X T (ed) Research on acupuncture, moxibustion, and acupuncture anaesthesia. Science Press, Beijing
120. Liang X 1979 Individual varitaion in acupuncture analgesia in rats in relation to 5-hydroxytryptamine (5HT) and endegenous opiate-like substances (OLS) in the brain. National Symposium on Acupuncture, Moxibustion and Acupuncture Anaesthesia, Beijing Paper No 507
121. Tang J, Liang X N, Zhang W Q, Han J S 1979 Acupuncture tolerance and morphine tolerance in rats. National Symposium on Acupuncture, Moxibustion and Acupuncture Anaesthesia, Beijing No 508 Full transcript in Chinese in Beijing Medicine 1:34–37, 1979
122. Han J S, Tang J, Huang B S, Zhang N H 1979 Acupuncture tolerance: The role of endogenous anti-opiate substances (AOS). National Symposium of Acupuncture and Moxibustion and Acupuncture Anaesthesia, Beijing Paper No 509
123. Zhang C L, Sun G D, Yan H Jet al 1986 Substance P: its analgesic effect and influence on caudate neuronal activity in conscious rabbits. In: Zhang X T (ed) Research on acupunctue, moxibustion, and acupuncture anaesthesia. Science Press, Beijing, p 388–396
124. Kenyon J N, Knight C J, Wells C 1983 Randomises double-blind trial on the immediate effects of naloxone on classical Chinese acupuncture therapy for chronic pain. Acupuncture and Electrotherapeutics Research 8: 17–24

FURTHER READING

Li P, Sun F Y, Zhang A Z 1983 The effect of acupuncture on blood pressure: the interrelation of sympathetic activity and endogenous opioid peptides. Acupuncture and Electrotherapeutics Research 8: 45–56
Li P, Lin S X 1981 Mechanism of inhibitory effect of electroacupuncture on noradrenaline hypertension. Acta Physiologia Sinica 33(4): 335–342
Zhou Z F 1980 Effect of intracerebral injection of clonidine or phentolamine on acupuncture analgesia in rabbits. Acta Physiologia Sinica 33:1–7
Xu S F, Cao X D, Mo W Y, Xu Z B, Pan Y Y 1987 The effect of the combination of drugs with acupuncture on analgesia efficacy. World Federation of Acupuncture Societies Conference, Beijing, p 215–217
Hokfelt T, Ljungdahl A, Terenius L, Elde R, Nilson G 1977 Immunohistochemical analysis of peptide pathways possibly related to pain and analgesia: enkephalin and substance P. Proceedings of the National Academy of Science USA 74(7): 3081–3085
Marx J L 1977 Analgesia: How the body inhibits pain perception. Science, February, p 471–473
Han J S, Terenius L 1982 Neurochemical basis of acupuncture analgesia. Annual Review of Pharmacology and Toxicology 22: 193–220
Ni L, Lu Z B, Liu D X 1984 Autoradiographic localisation of opiate receptors of the central nervous system in normal and acupunctured rabbits. Second National Symposium of Acupuncture, Moxibustion, and Acupuncture Anaesthesia, Beijing Paper No 643
Oliveras J L, Besson J M, Guilbaud G, Liebskind J C 1974 Behavioural and electrophysiological evidence of pain inhibition from midbrain stimulation in the cat. Experimental Brain Research 20: 32–44

6. Acupuncture as learning

It is obvious that acupuncture signals are mediated by a whole batch of neurotransmitters with a symphony of effects. And the yin yang dichotomy is valid even at this level. Some of the neurochemicals, such as the opiate peptides, serotonin, noradrenalin in the spinal cord (and via beta-receptors), and acetycholine are facilitatory to acupuncture analgesia. Others, such as the anti-opiate substances (including CCK-8), the catecholamines, especially noradrenalin in the brain (and via alpha-receptors), and gamma-aminobutyric acid (GABA) prove to be antagonistic to it. The strength of analgesia is determined by the balance of these factors within the central nervous system.

More complex neurotransmitter interrelationships than that between the opiates and serotonin described previously could easily account for some individual variations in the effectiveness of acupuncture analgesia or any other physiological responses to acupuncture. The variety of clinical studies, pharmacological manipulations, and neurological experiments in the literature bear witness to the range and sheer volume of studies. It is now becoming accepted in the West that acupuncture is capable of inducing widespread, substantial and permanent health responses. Varying experimental conditions, such as stimulation parameters, species of animal, environmental conditions, etc., can lead to contradictory results, but they certainly do not negate the trend of information.

There are experiments that direct attention to identifying drugs that potentiate the effect of acupuncture analgesia. For example, Xu Zhenbang in the Shanghai First Medical College confirmed that metoclopramide could ameliorate the analgesic response.[1] Metoclopramide suppresses dopamine, and encourages the availability of achetylcholine, due to its function as an anticholinesterase.[2,3] The application of drugs with little side effects in combination with the administration of acupuncture is providing promising results, particularly for the purpose of elevating the analgesic outcome and relieving some dependency on harsher anaesthetic drugs, especially important for patient groups at risk, such as the aged. Figure 6.1 outlines pharmacological manipulations that may be performed in order to enhance or suppress analgesia by altering the functional activity of specifically important neurotransmitters.

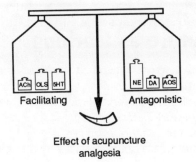

Facilitating   Antagonistic

Effect of acupuncture
analgesia

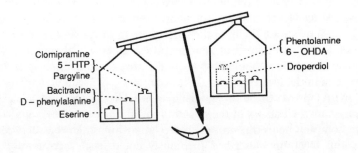

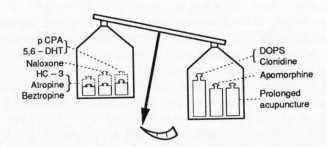

Fig. 6.1 The effect of altering the functional activity of central neurotransmitters on acupuncture analgesia. This diagram summarizes the main results of 7 years' study by Beijing scientists on the mechanism of acupuncture analgesia by the application of pharmacological manipulations.

Top: in ordinary conditions, the facilitating factors (ACh (acetylcholine), OLS (opiate-like substances), 5-HT (serotonin), etc.) and the antagonistic factors (NE (noradrenaline), DA (dopamine), AOS (anti-opiate substances), etc.) are driven into action simultaneously so that the effect of acupuncture analgesia is in the middle position.

Centre: the effect of acupuncture analgesia could be augmented by strengthening the functional activity of ACh, OLS and 5-HT and/or diminishing that of NE and DA.

Bottom: contradictory measures are taken to cut down the weight of the left side or to add to the weight of the right side which result in attenuation of the effect of acupuncture analgesia. (Reproduced with permission from Han J S, Tang J, Ren M F, Zhou Z F, Fan S G, Qiu X C 1980 Central neurotransmitters and acupuncture analgesia. American Journal of Chinese Medicine 8(4): 331–348.)

So far we have related most of the neurotransmitter research data to the nature and characteristics of acupuncture analgesia. It is beyond doubt that various transmitters act as mediators of the analgesic effect of acupuncture, and that alterations in the production and availability of these transmitters may also be reflected in more general physiological responses. The 20 to 30 minute build up of analgesia, its slow decay after cessation of stimulation and the phenomenon of acupuncture tolerance are all comprehensible in the neurotransmitter framework. However, what of the broader characteristics of physiological changes due to acupuncture?

As outlined in Chapter 2, acupuncture influences many physiological systems. However, there is not as yet a distinct link between the observation that increased frequency of treatment results in an increased therapeutic effect on the one hand, and altered neurological mechanisms on the other. Why, according to our previous research in acupuncture analgesia, should one treatment influence the next, even days apart? Not only does it appear to do so, but many researchers would argue, as does the whole empirical basis of Chinese medicine, that acupuncture mobilises a permanent change in some aspect of physiological behaviour, for example, in chronic headaches.[4]

Can acupuncture treat disorders by altering physiological patterns of behaviour, namely, changing physiological memory? The clinical characteristics of acupuncture, including the need for close repetition of treatment, certainly endorse this learning concept. Furthermore, it appears quite feasible that acupuncture could be perceived as a form of 'retraining' on a physiological level. To understand this properly, we need to explore further the physiological nature of memory.

Although there is still a lot to be learned about how memory operates, it is commonly believed that some actual anatomical, physiological or chemical change occurs in the synaptic junctions as a consequence of repetitive firing of these neurones and that these changes permanently facilitate the transmission of impulses at the synapses.[5] Synaptic change creates specific neuronal circuits through which signals pass with progressively greater ease the more frequently the same memory circuit is used. The more often the person *repeats the sensory experience*, the more established this neuronal circuit or 'memory engram' becomes. Rehearsal plays an extremely important role in the consolidation of memory engrams. At the most basic level, after stubbing one's toe on the same thing twice, one would soon learn to step to the side.

It is important to realise that memory extends far beyond simple recall of events and thoughts into the realm of physiological behaviour. Think, for example, of the instances where people may respond physiologically to certain situations, such as experiencing panic attacks whenever a particular sensory experience, for example, being with a large group of people, is repeated, or blushing in certain definable situations.

Not only does the sensory experience of acupuncture induce a range of neurotransmitter changes, but these changes themselves, if repeated frequently will also produce favoured neuronal circuits that will thereafter behave as a memory engram. It is possible that acupuncture treatments function as a learning experience, with each treatment representing a lesson whereby the body is physiologically taught to respond in a new fashion. Neuronal memory circuits are established that direct the patient toward new patterns of (healthier) physiological behaviour.

The concept that memory and learning may not be necessarily restricted to the brain, but rather be, at least, in part a generalised bodily reaction, is not unusual. Having spent 20 years searching for memory sites in the brain, Karl Lashley (1890–1958) concluded, 'I sometimes feel in reviewing the evidence on localisation of the memory trace that the necessary conclusion is that learning is not possible'.[6]

Lashley taught rats to perform in a maze and then removed specific parts of their brains. Although the surgery produced all kinds of deficits of movement, the animals still did not forget what they had learned; they could still find their way through the maze.

Various hormones have been linked to memory, including vasopressin (ADH), adrenocorticotrophic hormone (ACTH) and melanotrophin-stimulating hormone (MSH), to the extent that synthetic preparations of these hormones are being used to treat patients with memory loss. If these hormones are so crucial to memory, can learning go on outside the brain? Remember that opiate receptors are also located throughout many tissues including the gut and the peripheral blood vessels.

It is interesting also to note that the thalamus, a brain region with an important role in acupuncture, is thought to direct a person's attention to information in different parts of the memory storehouse. The thalamus itself is a brain region thought to be closely related to amnesia. Hence acupuncture, by influencing thalamic response, may well direct the body to recall healthy and normal physiological behaviour for which memory engrams should be well engrained in our bodies. Acupuncture itself may not be necessarily creating new physiological patterns of response, but rather reinforcing older established engrams of health to overcome patterns of illness, although the possibility of creation of new patterns should not be excluded.

Aside from the obvious characteristic that acupuncture treatments are beneficial if repeated in fairly close proximity, there are other characteristics that also mimic the neurological principles of learning. Habituation is where synapses (and hence a neuronal circuit) become desensitised after repeated stimulation. This occurs in order to avoid overcrowding the memory with unimportant sensory experiences or events. It is not unusual to note on occasion some degree of desensitisation to acupuncture after numerous treatments, and this may be one of the reasons why the ancient medical sages suggested a break in therapy after the initial standard course of 10 to 15 treatments. There is also some possible parallel here with the deterioration of analgesic response after three or so hours.

Sensitisation, the converse possibility, may also occur where the transmitter signal in the neuronal circuit becomes progressively stronger and may remain strong for hours, days, or even weeks, without further stimulation of the nerve terminal. Practitioners may describe the euphoria after treatment in this way, or it may offer some new angle to highly successful single treatments.

Finally it is important to note that people reinforce their learning and memory through reward. Sensory experiences associated with neither reward nor punishment are barely retained at all, and habituation to the stimulus develops. If a stimulus is associated with reward then the neurological response becomes progressively more intense each repetition. It is clear that encouragement and support and a positive attitude toward acupuncture treatment potentiates and amplifies the possible health response a patient may enjoy.[7] Just how much influence patients have on the outcome of their treatment as a consequence of whether they view it to be rewarding or not, is unknown.

Bearing in mind the wealth of research presented in the last decade it is interesting to note the conclusion of an earlier study (1979) appearing in Psychosomatic Medicine:[7]

Results are consistent with the view that acupuncture involves more than placebo factors, but the treatment appears to require a positive attitude of the recipient to potentiate its effect. (p 485)

Hence, there exists a possibility, different in a significant way to other theories so far proposed. This is that acupuncture therapy resembles a process of physiological relearning, and the neurological and hormonal changes that are usually reported during an acupuncture session represent only the immediate response.

Many of the clinical studies reviewed in Chapter 2 indicate that acupuncture is responsible for an element of more permanent change away from the pattern of an illness. This shift toward healthier physiological behaviour, may, in some cases, simply be a matter of activating the right trigger, but in most cases requires the persistent repetition of treatment. It appears that only under this constant encouragement do lasting changes occur.

Unless we admit some concept of learned behaviour, the neurohumoral research so far provides us only with an understanding of how acupuncture induces immediate responses, and not necessarily an understanding of how or why health has improved later. Yet the duration of the effect of acupuncture is as fundamental to its success and growth in popularity as are its short-term benefits, and if any theory is to be accepted by the scientific community it must also take into account this important characteristic.

Many explanations have been offered to explain the mechanisms of acupuncture, and these in turn have altered as awareness of acupuncture grew in the West. Each proposal usually had its weaknesses, which appeared after closer acquaintance with the practice of acupuncture and the breadth of its application. Although current neurophysiological understanding of acupuncture is very sophisticated and leaves no doubt as to the potential influence of acupuncture, even this theory needs to be refined or possibly even abandoned.

More importantly when we consider the hundreds of diseases to which the Chinese have applied acupuncture, it would appear incredible that this should have been developed totally by the hit or miss approach of empirical recording. Although that may well have a been a starting point, the scope of acupuncture required a theory that could lead to the development of the current variety of applications for acupuncture.

In fact acupuncture is being tested on new diseases and performing not unsuccessfully, implying that traditional theory holds some validity. We are able to use it to predict the possible applications of acupuncture. Not even the neurohumoral theory can as yet achieve this degree of success. And the use of modern neurophysiological concepts to predict the result of an acupuncture treatment would become so complex as to make the task impossible.

Conceptualizing acupuncture as a physiological learning process is important because it integrates the neurohumoral paradigm with the clinical characteristics of practice. So many other theoretical proposals have had to be discarded because precisely they fail to correspond with clinical reality.

The bioelectric theory is one that attempts to link the electromagnetic characteristics of the acupuncture points with myoelectric currents and neurohumoral changes, but as yet offers no great insight into the traditional Chinese theoretical constructions. The theory of acupuncture as a learning process provides a bridge between the neurohumoral paradigm and the short- and long-term nature of acupuncture therapy, but similarly it cannot be clearly related to traditional theory. There is a need for more research, nevertheless the outcome of the thousands of clinical and experimental studies over the last three decades is that acupuncture stands firmly as a valid, viable and often preferable form of treatment, and certainly not just for pain relief.

REFERENCES

1. Xu Z B, Pan Y Y, Xu S F, Mo W Y, Cao X D, He L F 1983 Synergism between metoclopramide and EAA. Acupuncture and Electrotherapeutics Research 8: 283–288
2. Karanth K S, Gurumadhra R S, Padma K T K, Guruswami M N 1981 Anticholinesterase activity of metoclopramide. Indian Journal of Medical Research 74: 125–128
3. Schulze-Delrien K 1981 Metoclopramide. New England Journal of Medicine 305: 28–33
4. Eriksson M B E, Sjolund B H, Nielzen S 1979 Long term results of peripheral conditioning stimulation as an analgesic measure of chronic pain. Pain 6: 335–347
5. Guyton A C 1982 Human physiology and mechanisms of disease, 3rd edn. Rigaku-Shoin/Saunders Publ., Philadelphia
6. Bergland R 1985 The fabric of mind. Penguin, Melbourne
7. Knox V J, Handfield-Jones C E, Shum K 1979 Subject expectancy and the reduction of cold pressor pain with acupuncture and placebo acupuncture. Psychosomatic Medicine 41(6): 447–486

Index

Surgical anaesthesia, 23–27, 39
  advantages/disadvantages, 27
  in children, 23–24
  duration, 26, 27
  ear points, 27
  effectiveness, 24
  individual characteristics and, 27
  manipulation of needles, 27
  onset of effect, 26, 27
  patient selection, 24–25
  pharmacological medication supplementing,
    17, 23–24, 25–26
  points selection, 27
  success rate, 23, 24
  types of surgery, 24, 25
Sympathetic nerve point, 6
Syringomelia, 61, 62

Tabes dorsalis, 61
Thalamus, 114, 117
  gate control theory and, 104–105
  memory response and, 130
Throat disorders, 24
Thromboangiitis obliterans, 20
Thrombocytopenic purpura, 36
Thyroidectomy, 24, 27
Thyrotropin-releasing hormone, 91
Tianzhu (Bl 10), 6
Time of needling, 9
Tinghui (GB 2), 42
Tolerance of acupuncture, 120–121
Tongue, 1, 2
Tonsillectomy, 23
Traditional Chinese medicine, 5–7
  diagnosis and *see* Diagnosis

integration with western science, 17–18
  pain and, 19–20
  causative factors, 20
  deficiency/excess classification, 20
Trigger spots, 59
Triglyceride levels, 34

Urinary bladder channel, 56
Urination control, 29
Urogenital conditions, 58

Vaccination, 38
Vasodilation/constriction, 9, 10
Viral infection, 94

Waiguan (SJ 5), 9
Weizhong (Bl 40), 6
White blood cell count, 29, 34–36, 43

Xi-Cleft points, 52
Xuanzhong (GB 39), 35, 38
Xuehai (Sp 10), 35

Yamen (Du 15), 34–35
Yangxi (Co 5), 32
Yinxi (Ht 6), 6

Zhishi (Bl 52), 39
Zhongwan (Ren 12), 58
Zusanli (St 36), 30, 31, 32, 33, 34, 35, 36, 37,
  39, 63, 117